He was still sitting on the floor, and tilted his head back to look at her.

It gave Mellie a new and strangely tantalizing view of his face, and her breath hitched in her chest as her gaze landed on and clung to his lips.

Delano had a mouth made for kissing—truly he did. It was full lipped but eminently masculine at the same time, with a natural upturn at the corners that took it from attractive into the "sinful" category.

The temptation to bend and put her mouth on his was almost overwhelming, and when the tip of his tongue slipped out to dampen his lower lip, a shudder of desire heated Mellie's skin.

No. No. No.

This wouldn't do, at all!

She spun on her heel and, in her haste, wobbled. Delano grabbed her leg, high up on her thigh, apparently trying to stabilize her balance. But what he did, instead, was make her gasp at the strength of his grip and the warmth of his palm evident through her scrubs.

Dear Reader,

Anyone involved with animal rescue is a hero to me. But if a rescuer happens to read this book, they'll probably laugh themselves silly at the idea of an island vet who somehow also has time to run a shelter. Believe me, having seen both veterinarians and rescue workers in the trenches, I was fully aware making my heroine, Mellie, juggle both occupations *and* find time to fall in love was stretching it!

Yet I wanted to highlight the world of animal rescue. It's not all cute kittens and puppies. It's hard, heartbreaking work that most of us wouldn't have the stomach for. The woman I've dedicated this book to had a dream of rescuing animals in Jamaica and, against all odds, made it a reality. Montego Bay Animal Haven is dear to my heart, and their Hiking with the Hooligans program is a must if you're visiting the island!

Rescuers suffer along with the animals, and mourn the ones they can't help or don't get to in time. In *The Vet's Caribbean Fling*, Delano and Mellie find love and healing in each other, and that's my wish for all the animals and their rescuers.

That love prevails, and heals us all.

Ann McIntosh

THE VET'S
CARIBBEAN FLING

ANN McINTOSH

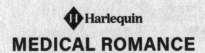

MEDICAL ROMANCE

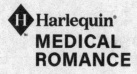

Harlequin®
MEDICAL ROMANCE

Recycling programs for this product may not exist in your area.

ISBN-13: 978-1-335-59554-6

The Vet's Caribbean Fling

Copyright © 2024 by Ann McIntosh

Harlequin Enterprises ULC
22 Adelaide St. West, 41st Floor
Toronto, Ontario M5H 4E3, Canada
www.Harlequin.com

Printed in U.S.A.

Ann McIntosh was born in the tropics, lived in the frozen north for a number of years and now resides in sunny central Florida with her husband. She's a proud mama to three grown children, loves tea, crafting, animals (except reptiles!), bacon and the ocean. She believes in the power of romance to heal, inspire and provide hope in our complex world.

Books by Ann McIntosh

Harlequin Medical Romance

Carey Cove Midwives

Christmas Miracle on Their Doorstep

Boston Christmas Miracles

The Nurse's Holiday Swap

Christmas with Her Lost-and-Found Lover
Night Shifts with the Miami Doc
Island Fling with the Surgeon
Christmas Miracle in Jamaica
How to Heal the Surgeon's Heart
One-Night Fling in Positano
Twin Babies to Reunite Them

Visit the Author Profile page at Harlequin.com.

To Tammy Browne Ogden, one of the kindest,
strongest, most amazing and beautiful women I
know. You make the world a better place
just by your existence (and I know a plethora of
animals that would wholeheartedly agree!).

CHAPTER ONE

THE CALL CAME at nine in the evening and, although not unexpected, it made Dr. Mellie Roscoe sigh.

"Snugums is nesting," Karyn Williams said, the fear in her voice obvious. "I think you should come."

Mellie bit back both another sigh and a sharp reply. Although she was fed right up with Karyn and her drama, the probability that her Yorkie, Snugums, might have problems delivering her pups was high.

Fighting annoyance, and keeping her voice as calm and level as possible, she said, "What's Snugums doing?"

"She's off her food—hasn't eaten today at all—and she's pawing around in the nursery, pulling all the towels and blankets together. I read that's a sure sign that she's about to give birth."

"Those are some of the indicators," Mellie agreed. "Is her belly really hard?"

"I'm not going to touch her to find out," Karyn all but wailed. "She growled at me earlier."

There was no way to stop herself from rolling her eyes, and Mellie was glad she wasn't face-to-face with the client.

"Well, you're going to have to be brave because

I want you to put her in the car and meet me at the clinic."

"Why can't you come here?" Panic laced the other woman's tone.

"Because if Snugums or the puppies are in distress, I want to be able to operate immediately. You're twenty minutes away from the clinic, and those minutes could make all the difference."

"If Snugums bites me when I try to get her in the car, I'm holding you responsible," was the unreasonable reply, followed by the unmistakable click of the phone being hung up.

It was only then that Mellie allowed herself to growl, and mutter a couple of curses. As she trailed into the kitchen to make herself a quick cup of coffee before going to meet Karyn, pairs of interested eyes followed her every move.

"Sorry, guys," she said to the three dogs, opening the back door so they could go out and do their business. "I'm heading right back out again to meet up with a princess and her Karyn, so make it snappy."

Under normal circumstances she'd be more sympathetic toward the other woman. After all, it was Snugums's first litter, but it was also an ill-advised one.

When Karyn had first approached Mellie about breeding the tiny bitch, Mellie had been blunt with her opinion.

"I wouldn't advise it, since any of the available males on St. Eustace will be related to her, and that is a risk in itself. Also, Snugums is rather small, and I can't think of a male smaller than she is, which is advisable when breeding a bitch of this size."

"I've never heard anything like that before," Karyn had scoffed, despite Mellie being the vet and Karyn a first-time pure-bred dog owner. Mellie was sure all Karyn was interested in was the idea of the money she could make from the puppies, which longtime breeders would say was a lot less than people thought. "Why would she need to be mated with a male smaller than she is?"

"Because if she mates with a male larger than she is, there's the risk that she can't deliver the puppies naturally. Then we'd have to do a Cesarian section."

Despite huffily saying she understood the difficulties, the next thing Mellie heard was that Snugums was in the family way.

It still rankled that Karyn would have ignored her advice. Having grown up with a hypercritical mother, it had taken a lot of hard work on Mellie's part to learn to speak up firmly. Once she'd mastered the art, it was a source of annoyance when people dismissed what she said.

"Don't worry about Karyn," Dr. Milo said, when Mellie brought it up with him. "I told her the same thing, so it wasn't just you she didn't listen to."

Worse, once it was confirmed Snugums was expecting, Karyn immediately went from cocky potential dog breeder to manic grandmother-to-be on steroids. Every few days, she'd brought Snugums to the clinic, quite sure that her "baby" was on death's door.

Even the ever-patient Dr. Milo, who Karyn insisted take care of Snugums, had begun to get testy about the whole situation. When the older vet had what he euphemistically called "a turn"—in reality a myocardial infarction—just a few days ago, Mellie had found herself in the unenviable position of taking over the Yorkie's care.

As if she didn't have enough on her plate, worrying about her mentor and friend's prospects of recovery, along with taking care of all the veterinary patients.

In fact, she'd just walked in the door after going across the island to drench a herd of cattle, which she'd only managed to get to after the clinic closed. Thankfully, being summer, she'd had enough light to get most of the herd done, and the farmer had brought out a standing light so she could do the last few.

Exhaustion dragged at her, but there was no way she would abandon a patient.

Thank goodness for her right-hand man, Johnny Luck, who'd fed all the animals after Mellie had called to let him know she'd be home late. Without the elderly man keeping an eye on things here at the shelter, she didn't know what she'd do.

After letting the dogs back in, Mellie poured the coffee into a travel mug. Sheba trotted over to come to stand beside her, big brown eyes looking up at her as if to ask, *You're going out again?*

Reaching down, Mellie scratched the little mongrel dog between her ears. "Sorry, girl. Mama's got another doggy to take care of."

Then, suppressing a yawn, she grabbed her tote and coffee, and went back out into the warmth and darkness of the Caribbean night to her car.

At that time of the evening it was only a ten-minute drive to the clinic, which was on a low hill on the road to downtown Port Michael, and Mellie spent the time mentally prepping for the upcoming delivery.

Since Dr. Milo's medical emergency, Mellie had been fretting about her ability to keep the Prospect Vet Clinic running by herself. Over the five years since she started working there, she and Dr. Milo had worked out a system that ran like clockwork.

They each had their own patients, but were always on hand to help each other out when needed. They'd shared the ubiquitous dogs and cats, but Dr. Milo did a lot of the large animal work, while he preferred to leave what he called the "exotic" animals to Mellie.

On St. Eustace, "exotic" was anything other than dogs, cats or farm animals, and consisted of rabbits, guinea pigs, birds and the occasional hamster—all well within Mellie's sphere of competence. So far no one had brought in a pet iguana, for which she was secretly grateful. She hadn't had any practice on a reptile since leaving vet school.

And even if before this last illness Dr. Milo had been showing definite signs of slowing down, but while Mellie had been handling more of the patients, he'd still been there to call on.

Now, as she drove through the night toward who knew what drama, Mellie couldn't help a shiver of apprehension. She'd be alone to deliver the pups—Karyn would be no help—and if she needed to do the C-section, it would be so much better to have someone there with her. The chances of finding a vet assistant willing and able to come back in to help were meager, at best. What if she lost the puppies? Or, worse, Snugums?

Then, on an inhale, she thrust her fear aside and tightened her grip on the steering wheel.

For the last couple of years, she'd been working and planning toward buying the seventy-year-old Dr. Milo out when he was ready to retire. Yes, it seemed as though that time might be coming sooner than she expected and, sure, she was finding the sudden plunge into being the only vet at the clinic harrowing. But in the final analysis, she was definitely ready if that was the way things panned out. The last four days had been chaotic, as she tried to fulfill all the obligations they'd committed to, but going forward things would smooth out.

She was sure of it.

Turning into the clinic parking lot, she drove around to the back and parked in her usual spot. The building exterior was lit by a number of lights, and the resident dogs in the kennels attached to the rear of the building let out a volley of welcoming barks as Mellie got out of the car.

Taking out her keys, she let herself into the kitchen/mudroom, and paused after pulling the door closed behind her.

"Who left on the light in the office?" she muttered, gazing at the triangle of light visible from the hallway, just as a shadow split it for a second, causing her heart to jump.

Frozen in place, her breath sawing in and out of her suddenly laboring lungs, she strained to hear anything from the office, anything at all, over the lingering barks and the rush of her own fear.

The dogs outside settled down somewhat, and in the sudden pocket of silence Mellie heard something like a bottle fall to the floor and a male voice grumble, as though in response.

And suddenly, ferociously, she wasn't afraid anymore.

She was livid.

How dare someone break into the clinic to rob it?

Without another thought, Mellie moved on near-silent, sneakered feet toward the corridor leading to the office, pausing only to pick up the machete used to trim the bushes around the building. Then she walked along to the door, and stepped into the office she and Dr. Milo shared.

"Who are you?" she barked. "And what do you think you're doing?"

The man, who was leaning into the medicine closet, jolted upright and spun around, whacking the side of his head on the open cupboard door so hard that even Mellie winced. But it didn't make her drop her aggressive stance—machete held up and out, as though prepared to do battle.

"What the hell?" The man stood glaring at her, rubbing his cheek. "You scared the daylights out of me."

"I'll do a lot more than that," Mellie retorted, lifting the machete a little higher and giving it a threatening swish. "How did you get in here, and what do you think you're doing?"

But a couple of thoughts hit her just then, shaking her assurance.

Firstly, the burglar was very large. At least four inches taller than her own five-foot-eight-inch height, very broad in the shoulders and overall muscular.

Taking him on in a fight wouldn't be easy.

Secondly, there was something vaguely familiar about him, although she knew, for a fact, she'd never seen him before. He was also—well—rather *dapper* for a burglar.

"Tall, dark and handsome" was such a cliché, but absolutely suited him.

With his neatly barbered hair, unwrinkled and expensive-looking polo shirt, "sleek and sophisticated" did too.

Sweat trickled down her back beneath her scrub top, as the man silently stared at her, his gaze shifting between her face and the machete. Instead of feeling scared or intimidated, Mellie was shocked by a rush of attraction, bordering on lust.

It took every ounce of determination she had

not to devour his delicious body with her eyes, and to remind herself he was some kind of criminal. By the time he finally spoke, Mellie was about to scream with the tension that had built up inside her.

"My name is Delano, and I'm Dr. Logan's son," he said calmly, his dark gaze flicking one more time to the machete before fixing on hers. "And, Dr. Roscoe, I'd suggest you put down that machete before you hurt yourself."

Over years of working with large animals—especially horses because of their almost psychic ability to read emotion and mood—Delano had learned to project nothing but tranquility.

Even when, like now, his instincts were screaming at him that this was a monumental moment, although he wasn't sure of what kind.

The woman standing in the doorway looked downright Amazonian—all bristled up and ready to defend herself and the clinic, no matter the cost.

And even from across the room, the keen edge on the blade in her hand was obvious.

He recognized her, of course, from the pictures his aunt and father had sent over the last few years. Dr. Mellie Roscoe, his father's junior associate and obvious favorite vet, present company not excepted. While they hadn't met before, Delano could only hope that someone had alerted her to his existence, and it wouldn't come as a shock.

Surely his father hadn't completely excised him from all conversation? Although there was always that possibility. For too many years to contemplate, since Delano was twelve and his mother had died, there had been a huge chasm between him and his father that felt too wide to cross.

Pushing that depressing thought away, and hoping his words would defuse the situation, he kept looking at her face and therefore saw exactly when his statement sank in.

Her eyes widened, and her mouth fell open slightly as her gaze scoured his face. Most importantly, the machete was lowered, so it hung by her side. But she didn't put it down.

Then, instead of apologizing, or offering any kind of friendly overture, her eyes narrowed and her top lip curled.

"Dr. Delano Logan…" She drew his name out, making the hair on the back of his neck rise at her laconic and somehow insulting tone. "Well, that's a bit of a surprise. What are you doing here?"

Taken aback all over again, Delano rubbed his still stinging cheek, wondering how to answer her rather rude question.

It shouldn't be a surprise to her that Delano had traveled to St. Eustace from Trinidad to be by his father's side after the elder Dr. Logan had a heart attack. Yet, she'd worked with his father for five years, and no doubt also knew Delano hadn't been back to his homeland for a very long time.

Not when Dr. Milo got an award from the chamber of commerce for his contributions to island life, nor when the Caribbean Veterinary Council honored him for his years of service. Delano had even missed his father's sixty-fifth birthday bash, although from the pictures it seemed almost the entire population of St. Eustace had been there.

He'd never even come back for any of the biennial dog shows his father organized in memory of Delano's mother, Iris, who'd had a passionate love of all canines.

She probably was also well aware of the problems within the Racing Commission back in Trinidad. Their press releases had been carefully uncommunicative, simply saying there had been some irregularities they needed to investigate, and that they were canceling race meets until further notice. While Delano knew the full story, he'd been asked not to speak about it, and hadn't; however, the rumors and gossip had flown and stung them all, even the innocent.

Just thinking about all those issues had guilt and shame crawling up in a heated wave from his chest into his throat, but he kept his face expressionless. There was another way to interpret her question regarding what he was doing there, and Delano quickly chose it.

"I'm looking for the broad-spectrum dewormers." Her eyebrows rose, and her head tilted to one side, as though his reply came as the surprise he'd hoped for. "For my dog, Baldur. I forgot to bring any for him, and he's due a dose now. I didn't want to wait until I got back to T & T, so Dad suggested I come down and get some from here. I walked down rather than bother driving such a short way."

She didn't respond immediately. Instead, she looked over her shoulder, and Delano saw a shaft of light that he thought was from an approaching vehicle travel across the wall outside the office.

"That'll be my patient coming in." Mellie glanced back at him, but there was no mistaking her dismissive tone. "Dewormer's on the right-hand side of the other cupboard."

Then, before he could say another word, she exited, thankfully taking the machete with her, and Delano took the first deep breath he'd been able to since he'd turned and seen her in the doorway.

His aunt had described Mellie Roscoe as a warm, fun, lighthearted person, who worked and played equally hard and got along well with everyone. Her pictures had shown a good-looking, smiling woman, almost invariably with her arm slung around some else's shoulders.

Somehow, now, he couldn't decide whether his aunt had misrepresented the vet's personality, or if it were he who brought out the worst in her. What he did have to acknowledge, though, was that she was far more beautiful in person than in those photos. Rich, brown skin stretched smooth and silky over an oval face. Full lips made him think of kissing even when she was frowning, and flashing light brown eyes seemed made for drowning in. In all honesty, their encounter had impacted him in ways he hadn't expected at all.

Even as she threatened him with a machete, he'd felt a definite thrill of attraction. One that was both unwanted and highly inadvisable. There was no room in his life for any kind of entanglement, especially not here in St. Eustace.

With a rueful headshake, Delano turned to the cupboard Mellie had indicated to hunt for the medication, all to a backdrop of muted conversation from one of the examination rooms. Thank goodness he only planned to be on the island for a couple of weeks, so he wouldn't be too tempted to try and figure Mellie Roscoe out.

"Hey."

He hadn't heard her come back to the door, and only narrowly missed whacking his head again when he spun around to face her.

"What?"

"Make yourself useful, and help me do an ultrasound on a dog? She may need a Cesarean section and I need someone to keep her calm while I take a look at the puppies' placement and size."

She still didn't look friendly. In fact, she looked as though asking him was the last thing she wanted to do, which made Delano feel even more annoyed. Let her handle her business on her own, then.

"Sure," he heard himself say, contrary to his thought. He even threw in one of his best, most charming smiles for good measure. "I can do that."

From her little snort—which sounded suspiciously like disgust—you'd think he'd refused instead. And Delano found himself smiling as he followed her out of the office and into the examination room.

This just might be fun, after all.

CHAPTER TWO

Delano Logan.

Here in Port Michael, at the Prospect Clinic, acting as though he somehow belonged.

No. As though he *owned* the place.

He even had the nerve to be cheerfully accommodating when she asked for his help, and charming enough to turn Karyn Williams's head. There'd been no mistaking the double take and kittenish behavior the other woman had immediately exhibited on being introduced to the handsome vet. And even though neither Mellie nor Delano was really paying her any attention, Karyn was droning on behind them, clearly trying to attract his attention.

Worst of all, while he was leaning over the examination table, whispering sweet nothings to an adoring Snugums and Mellie shaved the Yorkie's belly, he smelled like a dream...

A very naughty dream, in fact.

The last time she'd been attracted to a man of this type, in this way, the result had been embarrassment, heartbreak, financial devastation and a protracted lawsuit aimed at getting restitution.

There was no way her heart should be thumping with awareness, or that her focus wanted to stray away from her patient to the man beside her.

The unwanted physical reaction to him was just one more reason to be angry with him; not that she needed additional stimulus. While her emotions about his sudden advent into her life were confused, none of them were positive.

As she got the ultrasound machine set up, she tried to get her feelings under control but kept cycling back to the crux of the matter, which didn't help in her effort to calm down.

Dr. Milo meant the world to her. He'd given her a spot in his clinic when she'd desperately needed a job, on just her father's assurance that she knew what she was doing. His illness had affected her profoundly—the same way, she suspected, as it would have had it been her own father. She knew Milo must be over the moon to have his son come home to be with him at a time like this, and under normal circumstances she would be too.

But who could trust Delano and his motives when he'd ignored his father for years?

When he'd turned up only after his job as a race-course veterinarian seemed in jeopardy?

Coincidence? Happenstance?

Mellie didn't think so, and it made her blood icy to think of him causing his father additional hurt, should it come out that he was simply here with an eye to the main chance.

But she also had to admit she felt hurt by the fact Dr. Milo hadn't even let her know his son was back on the island. She thought they were closer than that.

Hard not to feel rejected, like the other brother in the story of the Prodigal Son. The one who'd kept on the straight and narrow—was dependable—and couldn't understand what the fuss was about when the wastrel son came home.

There was, she thought, a lesson in there somewhere, but she was too busy just now to figure it out.

As she pressed the transducer into Snugums's distended belly, her gaze on the monitor, she was desperately trying to ignore the warm, spicy scent emanating off Delano's skin. Then, as she shifted the transducer, her heart did a little dip toward her stomach, and Delano let out a soft grunt.

"What? What is it?"

Apparently Karyn had been paying some attention to what they were doing, and had picked up on their reactions. Mellie took a deep breath, knowing if she exhibited any of the anxiety shivering along her spine, Karyn would probably lose it.

"In my opinion, the puppies' heads are too big to pass through the birth canal." There was no way to soft-soap it. "If we let Snugums try to deliver them vaginally, we'd be risking both her life and the lives of the pups. I'm suggesting I perform an emergency C-section, rather than take the risk."

Karyn immediately turned and asked Delano, "What do you think I should do?"

Mellie raised her eyebrows, but stayed silent. It would be instructive to see how Delano responded.

"I think," he said slowly, "you should listen to your vet."

"No." Karyn swept her carefully straightened hair back over her shoulder and gave her head a toss. "You're a vet too. I want to hear your opinion, before I make a decision."

Remember you're a professional.

Mellie's jaw clicked with the pressure she put it under, and she turned her back on the other woman, firmly keeping the words fighting to come out behind her teeth.

It wasn't the first time someone had tried to do an end run around her, usually appealing to Dr. Milo rather than listening to what Mellie said. But no matter how often it happened, it never failed to rile her up. After all, casual misogyny wasn't confined to men. Some of the worst she'd experienced had been at the hands of women.

"I don't have an opinion," Delano said, his voice quiet and deep. "I'm not your dog's primary veterinarian. Dr. Roscoe is, and she's given her diagnosis."

Karyn seemed set to continue arguing, but just then Snugums whimpered.

"Oh, all right, do the C-section, but I'm holding you responsible—"

"Yes. Yes. I know." Fed up, Mellie couldn't stop herself from interrupting the familiar refrain. "If you'll wait in the reception area, I'll get the paperwork together for you to sign."

Thankfully, Karyn stomped off, and Mellie let

out a long exhale. The part of her that appreciated Delano supporting her, rather than taking the chance to undermine her, insisted that she thank him, but she knew it would sound grudging, so she didn't.

"Can you stay with Snugums for a little longer?" she asked instead. "I need to see if I can locate one of the vet techs, and print out the waiver for Karyn to sign."

"Will any of your techs be available on a Friday night, at almost ten o'clock?" he asked in response. "I can assist, if you need me to. I'll just need to call the house and let them know what's happening."

His mentioning Dr. Milo squelched any softer feelings Mellie might have started to develop toward him, and she frowned. But as she was about to refuse his offer, Delano continued.

"And before you ask, I do small animal work in Trinidad too, not just work with horses."

"I actually wasn't going to ask that," she huffed, picking up Snugums and placing her back in her carrier, where she'd be safe for the moment. Turning to face Delano, she crossed her arms. "However, I was going to suggest that your father is probably looking forward to you coming back to the house to spend time with him."

The expression that crossed his face was fleeting, and she wasn't sure exactly what the emotion was—only saw the way the corners of his mouth turned down slightly. Then he smiled and shrugged.

"He was already getting ready for bed when I

left. Aunt Eddie will still be up, though. She's a night owl."

Somehow, although she still wanted to refuse his offer of help, now she felt as though she couldn't, and those conflicting impulses made her huff out an annoyed breath.

"All right," she said, aware she was more miffed with herself than him, but knowing it probably didn't sound that way. "Let's get this done."

It had been a while since Delano had performed a C-section on such a small animal, but he remembered the routine well. You had to move quickly, not just for the health of the dam but also so the anesthetic didn't get to the puppies, or at least their exposure was minimized.

Because of his lack of familiarity with the operating theater, which hadn't been set up this way when he left, he felt a bit useless when it came time to prepare. However, Mellie proved patient and organized, directing him to where he could find all they needed in her brisk, if cool, way.

"Do you feel comfortable intubating?" she asked. They'd already inserted the IV and done a preliminary scrub of the site. It had also been decided that she'd perform the surgery, of course, while he took care of the pups once they'd been removed from the uterus.

"Yes."

Mellie took one last look at everything laid out,

as though going through a mental checklist, and then gave a decisive nod.

"Okay, let's go."

She administered the anesthetic, then they secured Snugums to the table. Once Delano had intubated the dam, he had a few moments to watch as Mellie began the operation. Her movements were deft, displaying both confidence and competence, which weren't always mutually inclusive. The technique she used was different from the one he generally favored, but wasn't unfamiliar to him, and soon she had exteriorized the first uterine horn and the uterine body. After packing the abdominal cavity with moistened laparotomy pads, she incised into the uterine body and used scissors to extend the cut.

Then the first puppy was extracted and handed to him, and he was too busy to look over Mellie's shoulder. He had to work quickly to free each pup from the amniotic sack, clamp their umbilicus, clean them up, suction their noses and mouths, and assess their conditions. Thankfully, each of the first three began breathing on their own and went into the incubator. The fourth, however, needed a dose of doxapram, but quickly thereafter started breathing without Delano having to do chest compressions or mouth-to-mouth resuscitation.

"Four healthy puppies," Delano commented, ligating the last pup's umbilicus and disinfecting the stump.

"No thanks to the owner," Mellie muttered. "I warned Karyn about mating Snugums, but…"

Her voice tapered off, ending on an exhale. She was closing the skin in a subcuticular pattern with dissolvable microfilament, so there would be no need to have the stitches removed later. It also stopped the puppies sucking on external sutures and aggravating the wound site.

"All's well that ends well," he said absently, which earned him a snort from Mellie.

"Don't jinx us now," she replied, with the first hint of humor he'd heard from her. "Let's get Snugums up and taking care of her pups before we pat ourselves on the back."

"Are you going to send Snugums home, or keep her under observation here until she comes out from under the anesthetic?"

Mellie sent him a sideways, one-eyebrow-up glance.

"Do you honestly think Karyn will be a suitable supervisor?" She gave another snort, and a brisk headshake. "I'll take them home with me and keep them until morning."

Was that weariness in her voice? Dad had made a point of saying that Mellie had somehow been able to take care of everything at the clinic since his heart attack, despite it usually being two of them working. If Mellie took the Yorkie and her pups home, she'd have to stay up a minimum of two hours more, to make sure the anesthetic had worn off completely and Snugums didn't inadvertently hurt her puppies.

Mellie gave Snugums the reversal shot, and then

removed the endotracheal tube. Delano helped her remove the restraints, and then asked, "Where do you want her?"

"Over in the recovery cage," she replied, gesturing to one of the top two built-in kennels against the wall.

It didn't take more than a moment to do as directed, but when he asked about reuniting the puppies with their mother, Mellie said to leave them in the incubator for a while longer.

"I want to keep an eye on all of them before I put them in with her." She paused beside the incubator and looked at the pups, a little smile tipping her lips. "They're so tiny, even Snugums could do them an injury if she were to step on them."

"Like tiny little sausages," Delano agreed, drawing an abbreviated chuckle from her.

After stripping off her gloves and washing her hands, she rubbed at the back of her neck as she turned to him, and he was sure the bags under her honey-colored eyes were from exhaustion.

"Why don't you let me take them back to Dad's?" He wasn't sure where the idea came from, but it seemed a good one. "I slept on the flight coming over, so I'm not tired at all."

"No." Her tone was abrupt, snappish, and her lips tightened for an instant before she continued, "I can manage."

Obviously she didn't want his help, but something prodded Delano to persist.

"Really, it's no problem."

She turned from where she was standing by the sink, and glared at him.

"I said I don't need your help taking care of Snugums and her puppies. Now, excuse me while I go and inform Karyn of what's happened. You can go home now."

Stung, and feeling as though she'd dismissed him like a pesky gnat, Delano couldn't resist taunting her in return.

"What? No, *Thank you for your help and kind offer, Delano*? Just, *Be gone, foul fiend*?"

Whatever response he was expecting, it wasn't for her to not even miss a beat on her way to the door, and he was beginning to wonder if she'd even reply when she opened the door and paused for an instant.

Without even looking his way, she simply said, "Exactly. By the way, that's not even a real quote from Shakespeare."

And having had the last word, she continued on her way, leaving him shaking his head in her wake.

CHAPTER THREE

DESPITE NOT GETTING to bed until after one, Mellie was up and checking on Snugums and her puppies by six the following morning. The Yorkie dam had taken longer than expected to shake off the effects of the anesthesia the night before and, once she had, at first showed little interest in her pups. Eventually Snugums started sniffing and licking the puppies, and didn't object when Mellie got them suckling in a nice little row.

"Don't get used to the organization," she muttered to Snugums. "It won't be long before they're all over the place, driving you nuts."

The little dog just looked up at her, before putting her head down, as though exhausted. Thankfully, that had signaled Mellie's chance to go shower and then go to bed.

Heavy-eyed and yawning, she was happy to see everything was fine—none of the pups bleeding from their tied-off umbilical cords, no sign of infection in the mother. Snugums couldn't be coaxed to leave the pups to go outside, and Mellie didn't try to force her. In fact, it was a bit of a relief. With all the other animals around, it was better and more sanitary the Yorkie stay sequestered in the powder room until Karyn came to pick her up.

After letting Sheba, Smudge and Ursa out, Mellie shuffled into the kitchen to make herself a much-needed cup of coffee. Outside she could hear Johnny Luck whistling as he released the other dogs from their kennels and started his day too. Between the two of them, they'd feed and water all the animals, clean the kennels, stable and fowl coop, and administer any medication necessary.

Thank goodness she didn't need to tackle the pigsty today.

As used to it all as she was, Mellie couldn't help contemplating the day ahead with dread brought on by exhaustion. She'd also been too tired the night before to stew on the latest drama unfolding in her life, but now that she was awake it all flooded back.

Delano Logan was charming, handsome and smooth, and Mellie didn't trust him farther than she could throw him. Although strong and fit, she didn't think she could even pick him up, so while the thought of tossing him like a caber was a pleasant one, it was firmly in the realm of imagination.

Mellie considered herself something of an expert on untrustworthy males. How could she not be, after her experience with Kyle? She'd learned the hard way that charm and winning smiles often went along with selfishness and questionable, or lacking, morals.

No one could have told her anything bad about Kyle back when they were together and make her believe it. He'd been sweet, winning and loving. He hadn't showered her with gifts, but had done little things to make her feel treasured. She'd been charmed enough to buy into a fantasy of happy-ever-after, which included her moving to Miami with him and providing the downpayment on a fixer-upper house. She hadn't been able to go on the title, because she didn't qualify for a mortgage, but Kyle had assured her that once they were married, it would all be legally taken care of.

Kyle had also convinced her to hold off finding a steady job. She'd had some experience working in her stepfather's construction firm, so she'd spent most of her time doing repairs to the house, getting it close to completion.

Then it had all fallen apart.

He'd gone behind her back and sold the house.

At Christmas, no less.

And that's when she'd found out it had all been one big scam.

Homeless and broke, she'd learned the hard way never to put her future into anyone else's hands. And the way things were shaping up with Dr. Milo and Delano, she couldn't help thinking she was heading right back into a similar situation.

That Delano was a threat to everything she'd worked for.

Last night her first thoughts had been for Dr. Milo, who might be hurt by his son no matter what Delano ended up doing. Now, however, Mellie had to admit to herself that her true feelings weren't entirely selfless. She was also worried on her own behalf.

Almost three years ago, Dr. Milo had spoken to her about the fate of his practice when he retired.

"Once, I'd hoped Delano would come home and take it over," he'd said, trying to sound matter-of-fact, but just sounding stilted and a little sad. "But now I realize I have to accept that he's settled in Trinidad and has no plans to ever live here again."

"So what's plan B?" she'd asked, holding her breath, hope swirling in her chest like dog hair in the groomer's drying room.

"Well," he'd replied, dragging the word out. "Hopefully I'll find someone willing to buy me out, and I can retire with a little nest egg."

She'd let out a long, silent exhale, before saying, "If that's the case, Doc, I'd like right of first refusal."

Dr. Milo had smiled then, his eyes starting to twinkle, and he'd replied, "Okay."

With that one word of agreement, Mellie had seen her future clearer than she'd ever been able to before.

She'd always hoped to have her own clinic one day, but just then—here on the island she'd come to call home—she could actually envision it.

But suddenly, now, when his job seemed to be hanging in the balance and his father might just be about to retire, here comes Delano sniffing around.

And threatening to make all of Mellie's hard work be for nothing.

Truthfully, she felt horrible even thinking that way. After all, it was a good thing that Delano was here to be with his father during the older man's illness. But no matter how she looked at it, Mellie could see no upside for herself.

If Delano decided to stay, she had no doubt Dr. Milo would hand the clinic over to him without hesitation, ignoring all that Mellie had put into it. Keeping her to an associate position, rather than an owner.

If Dr. Milo recovered enough to come back to work, and Delano went back to Trinidad, the visit might give Dr. Milo hope that his son could be convinced to eventually take over.

The final analysis, she decided, was she couldn't trust Delano to do right by his father or, if his decision affected her, do right by her either.

With that depressing and rage-inducing thought in mind, she took a sip of her coffee before going to change the cat litter and fill the feeding bowls.

Once that was done, she took the rest of her now lukewarm drink out into the yard so as to get to work.

By seven thirty she'd just finished feeding the pigs, Jane and Bingley, and was standing by their pen when Dr. Milo called. After a deep breath, she answered.

"Dr. Milo. How're you feeling today?"

"Good-good, Mellie." She could hear the joy and good humor in his voice. "I'm ready to go dancing, but Eddie won't let me."

Mellie snorted with laughter. "Glad to hear that

your sister is keeping you under control. You can't be trusted to stay quiet, the way the doctors want."

"Cho, them doctors just beating up their gums." He chuckled, then continued, "I hear you met Delano last night."

The change of subject caught her off guard, and Mellie had to take a steadying breath before she replied, "Yes. We surprised each other at the clinic."

"If I'd known he was coming, or that you'd be at work at that hour of the night, I'd have called to let you know, but he just turned up around dinnertime. Gave me a bit of a shock, can I tell you?"

Ridiculous to surprise a man who'd had a heart attack like that. Another indication in her books that Delano might just be a narcissist. Or a socio-path.

Keeping her dislike out of her voice took some effort, but she thought she did credibly well when she replied, "You must have been happy to see him."

"I was. And I'm sure you were happy for the help with the C-section on Snugums Williams."

"I was glad for the extra hands," she admitted grudgingly. "At least two of those puppies' heads were bigger than Snugums's pelvic canal. She'd have never been able to deliver them naturally."

"Delano said he offered to bring them all here and keep an eye on them for you, but you refused." Was that a hint of a reprimand in the older doctor's voice? It seemed as though it was, as he said, "You should have taken him up on the offer. I wouldn't have minded at all."

"It was no problem," she lied, keeping her voice light. "I put them in the powder room, away from all the other animals, and as soon as I get off the phone with you, I'm calling Karyn to come get them and take them home."

"Well, with everything you've been having to do since I've been ill, I'd have preferred you taking the opportunity to get some rest, but you know your own mind. What do you have going on today? I know there's no spay and neuter clinic this week, but are you giving a talk anywhere?"

Since starting her small animal shelter, Mellie had networked like crazy, getting sponsorships so she could offer low-cost and, in some cases, free spay and neuter days. They, along with educational outreach programs, would hopefully go a long way to curb the incidents of unwanted puppies and kittens as well as stray dogs and cats roaming the streets.

"No. I don't have anything planned today." Never had she been more relieved to have something of a free day, once all the animals were taken care of. But she didn't say so, knowing Dr. Milo was already stressing over the amount she was working.

"When is the next spay and neuter clinic?"

Wondering why he was asking, she replied, "In two weeks, in Grand Harbor."

"Well, I've asked Delano to help out while he's here—at the clinic and anything else I can't manage—so put him down for a shift. He can run the obedience classes too."

Biting back the sharp retort that rose to her lips, Mellie took a moment to get herself under control.

"Thanks, but you know I have things well in hand, right? Why don't you take the opportunity to spend time with your son, instead of farming him out like a workhorse?"

"Yes," was the decisive answer. "I know I can depend on you, but I don't want Delano sitting around all day, doing nothing. And if he doesn't take over the obedience classes, the dogs will forget all they've learned."

It sounded like Dr. Milo was clutching at straws, and although Mellie wanted to argue, she also didn't want to upset the older man.

So, suppressing a sigh, she said, "If he's serious about it, tell him to come into the clinic on Monday. I'm sure we can find something for him to do."

And there was no mistaking the satisfaction in Dr. Milo's voice as he finished the conversation and hung up.

As she punched the telephone screen to disconnect the call, Mellie muttered a string of curses.

The entire situation was going from bad to worse.

Delano retreated into the house without his father knowing he had even been there, and wandered toward the kitchen with Baldur, his Doberman pinscher, shadowing his steps. Hearing his father say he didn't want Delano sitting around the house doing nothing all day should be infuriating but, in reality, it just confirmed what Delano already suspected.

His father didn't want to spend more time with him than he had to.

Who could blame him? Having to see the person responsible for your beloved wife's death day in and day out must be excruciating. Which is why Delano had stayed away so long.

The guilt and sorrow that always flooded him whenever he'd thought about returning to St. Eustace filled him again now. In the past he'd used it as an excuse not to come home, but when he'd heard about his father's heart attack, he knew he had put off returning for too long.

Delano loved his dad, irrespective of how his father felt about him, and there was no way he'd shirk his responsibility of love just to avoid his own pain.

If all his father wanted was someone to take over his myriad occupations, and that would help keep him calm and well, then that was what Delano would do.

Although, he couldn't help wondering how the icy Mellie Roscoe was going to take having to interact with him all the time.

She'd made it absolutely clear that, like his father, she didn't want him around. But while his father's attitude made him sad, the thought of tweaking Mellie's tail was somehow highly amusing. Softening her up, charming her in whatever way he could, would give him a sorely needed distraction.

He was so lost in thought he almost ran into Aunt Eddie as she came out of the kitchen.

"Where you going?" she asked, putting her arms akimbo. "You just finished breakfast. Don't be going into my kitchen to mooch."

Delano couldn't help laughing and teasing his father's sister. "Cho-man, Aunt Eddie. But I hungry."

Her face softened into a fond smile. "You know how long I've been waiting to hear you say those words to me again? Come. Let me see what's in the fridge."

Slinging his arm around her shoulders, Delano confessed, "I'm not really hungry, Auntie. I just said so to annoy you. I could use another cup of coffee, though, but I can get that myself."

"Let me spoil you a little, at least today," she said, tiptoeing to kiss his cheek. "Tomorrow you can start looking after yourself."

Sitting at the kitchen table, Delano watched his aunt smoothly moving around the room, his heart swelling with love for the woman who'd moved in and helped raise him since he was a teen.

"So, you had a baptism by fire, eh? Delivering puppies on your first day back home."

"It was a surprise," he replied. "But not as much of one as being accosted by a machete-wielding woman out of the blue."

Aunt Eddie chuckled, shaking her head as she got the coffee maker going. "That Mellie is something else, isn't she? A real firecracker. Hard worker too.

You know she has an animal shelter at her home, don't you?"

"I don't think you mentioned that to me." Even if his aunt had, it wouldn't have meant too much to him. Everything about his homeland—with the exception of his father and aunt—had felt way too distant to be of much interest.

"When she came here, her father, Charlie—you remember Charlie Roscoe? He's a friend of your father—he gave her the old farm cottage he'd inherited from his uncle to live in. It sits on two acres, and once Mellie started taking in strays, everyone was bringing all kinds of beasts. Everything from cats and dogs to pigs and a turkey. She had to figure out a way to keep it going, so she turned it into a nonprofit, and gets donations to help run the place."

"Ahh…"

"She was saying it's getting crowded now, and she's contemplating buying a piece of land she's seen for sale, a bit farther up Long Hill, but I think she's waiting to see how things pan out first."

Aware that his aunt was looking at him out of the corner of her eye, Delano raised his eyebrows, and asked, "Things? What things you mean, Aunt Eddie?"

"Well, like whether you plan to stay here and take over your father's place at the clinic, or not."

The shock of her words left him speechless for a long moment. Is that what everyone was thinking, that because of the trouble back in Trinidad, he was looking to come back to St. Eustace and take over the clinic? His physical reaction to the thought made him have to swallow as a sickly sensation tickled the back of his throat.

Then he got himself under control and, well aware of his aunt's eagle eyes on him, he forced a smile and shook his head.

"If that's the case, then you should let her know I don't plan to do any such thing."

And, although he really wanted to walk away, he stayed where he was, pretending not to notice the frown his aunt sent him from across the room.

CHAPTER FOUR

MELLIE CAME UP with a plan of action to deal with Delano Logan at work.

Cool, calm and distant were the bywords, but there was no way to know beforehand just how difficult he would make it to stick to her guns.

The damned man was a force of nature: full of smiles, jokes and the kind of casual charm that no one seemed immune to.

Except Mellie, who was determined not to succumb.

He came strolling in on Monday morning, his red and rust Doberman, Baldur, heeling by his side despite being off leash.

"Good morning."

Just the cheerfulness of his voice made the hair stand up on the back of her neck, and Mellie suppressed a shiver. Looking up from the paperwork she was doing before her first patient, she nodded.

"Morning." In contrast, she made her voice sound brisk and impersonal. "Will you be bringing your dog with you to work every day? Is he sociable?"

Delano looked down and scratched the Dobe on the top of its head.

"Baldur? He's very chill. Not nosy or aggressive,

and since I take him for long runs each morning, he'll be happy to spend most of the day lazing about in here." With a hand signal, he released Baldur from his heel, and the Dobe gave a vigorous shake and started investigating the room. "He doesn't mind strangers, but usually chooses not to engage with people."

"Really?" Mellie retorted, trying not to laugh, since Baldur had stopped beside her and plopped his head into her lap, his ears lying back almost flat and his golden eyes beseeching pets. There was no way to ignore such a winning appeal, and Mellie happily gave in. "Yes, I can see how aloof he is."

Delano snorted. "Traitor, making me look like a liar right out the gate."

There were several thoughts that popped in her head, but Mellie kept them to herself. No need to start the day off on a sour note.

Instead, she asked, "Why did you decide to crop his ears? He's not a show dog, is he?" She didn't try to hide her disapproval, but Delano didn't seem to mind.

"No." Delano dropped into the other office chair and spun it to face her. "His conformation isn't right. He's too long for his height, and his ears sit too low, but he's actually a rescue, of a kind. His original owner thought he'd make some money off him if he won dog shows, and once he realized that wasn't going to happen, he wanted to put him down. I took him, instead."

Horrified, Mellie bent to hug Baldur. "I'm glad.

He's lovely, no matter what anyone else—or the conformation standard—says."

"I agree," Delano said, easily. "If I'd had him from a pup, I wouldn't have cropped his ears, and he'd have a tail too, if I'd had any say in the matter. Thankfully, it seems more people are turning away from those types of cosmetic changes."

Giving the Dobe another squeeze, Mellie replied, "It's illegal in some countries, but getting animal-based laws passed is an uphill battle in so many others."

Perhaps the embrace was too much for Baldur, because, after giving Mellie a lick, he eased out of her arms and lay down under her desk, taking up all the space where her feet should go.

Feeling as though her interaction with the dog had already undermined her determination to keep Delano at arm's length, Mellie made her tone cool again as she said, "We should discuss what you're interested and willing to do while you're here."

"Oh, I'll do anything," he replied, twisting his chair back and forth as though unable to keep still. "Just tell me what you need."

That felt like a completely loaded suggestion, and Mellie had to force herself not to let her mind wander down a dangerous and delicious path. Clearing her throat, she leaned back in her own chair and narrowed her eyes at him.

"Usually, your dad takes the larger animals and I do a lot of the small animal work, but I don't think we have anything with cattle or horses on the schedule just now. So why don't you see patients, while I check up on the animals we're monitoring here? Later, we can alternate with the patients. If you're comfortable with that, I'll tell Jackie, the receptionist, that she can book additional appointments. We'd cut back this week because of your dad being ill."

"Sounds good," he said in that easy way, as he put one ankle up onto the opposite knee, apparently about to settle in for a chat. "Aunt Eddie tells me you have an animal shelter? How many animals do you have?"

"A lot," she replied, knowing she was being abrupt and borderline rude. Getting up, she shuffled the papers into a neat pile, and said, "I'm heading down to the kennels, and you should probably take some time to figure out where everything is. The vet techs will help you."

Then, trying to ignore the way her skin felt tight and hot, and the tantalizing scent of his cologne lingering in her nostrils, she walked out as quickly as she could without seeming as though she was running away.

Although, since she'd effectively taken herself off to another part of the clinic, it did kind of feel like she was fleeing Delano's company.

There was something about his dark, twinkling eyes and the hint of a dimple in his cheek when he smiled that made her heart beat faster and threw her into a state of confusion.

And her determination to ignore Delano's presence as much as possible turned out to be almost impossible.

The first three days they had such an influx of clients—both old and new—that they were kept jumping. Even Mellie's best friend, Amity, was amongst the crowd.

"You'd believe every puss, dog and hamster suddenly needed to be examined," Mellie said to Amity on the phone after the second day. "I think we've had every female animal owner we've ever seen, and some new ones too, coming in once word got out that Delano was working at the clinic. Including you."

Amity just giggled. "Kitty-Puss needed her medication. Did you want her to run out?"

"Usually you call and ask me to bring it home for you, but this time you just had to come and pick it up yourself, eh?"

"Of course." Amity was still snickering. "After the way you'd been going on about him being here, I had to judge him for myself. I couldn't trust you to be impartial."

"For goodness' sake. You're as annoying as he is."

"Are you sure he's annoying you?" Amity asked, and Mellie knew if she could see her friend, there'd be a devilish sparkle in her eyes. Amity was such a brat. "Or is he turning you on? He's hot like fire!"

Mellie wished she could disagree, but her friend was right and they both knew it. And Mellie found herself more and more fascinated by Delano as the days passed. Although they mostly worked separately, in between patients their paths crossed continuously.

Then, at lunchtime on Wednesday, they had an existing canine patient, Rufus, come in having been hit by a car. Unfortunately Cecil, the surgical tech, was out of the clinic. When Mellie called and found out he was actually on the other side of Port Michael, she realized they couldn't wait for him to come back.

"Call the patients that have appointments right after lunch," she told Jackie, the receptionist. "Tell them we have an emergency and might be running late. They can come in and wait or reschedule."

Then she and Delano rushed the large mongrel down to surgery.

After they'd sedated Rufus and started hydrating him with Lactated Ringer's, they were able to examine him thoroughly and staunch the bleeding. X-rays showed the extent of the damage to his right hind leg, and Delano whistled.

"Yeah," Mellie said, pointing to the image. "With this amount of damage to the tibia and fibula, and the break in the femur…"

She trailed off, contemplating what to tell the dog's owner. They certainly could repair the damage but, as bad as it was, it would be an expensive operation. The procedure would involve painstakingly rebuilding the bones, pinning the repairs in place, and affixing the pins to external plates. She wasn't sure the elderly Mr. Brixton would be able to afford the surgery, or provide the dog with the appropriate aftercare. Yet, she also knew how attached the gentleman was to Rufus.

"What are you thinking?" Delano asked, as Mellie stripped off her gloves and tossed them into the garbage. He was lightly stroking Rufus's head, and Mellie found her gaze following the slow, tender movement of his fingers for a moment.

Then she sighed, and looked him in the eyes.

"I'll get Jackie to calculate the cost of surgery, but I think both poor Rufus and Mr. Brixton would be better off if we amputate the leg. The aftercare will be less extensive and the bill would be far less."

"Agreed," he replied. Then he turned toward the autoclave, as though ready to set out the necessary surgical instruments. "Just let me know what he decides, and let's get this fellow sorted out as quickly as possible. I'll keep an eye on him and watch for signs of internal bleeding while you deal with the owner."

She shouldn't feel relieved just because Delano agreed with her diagnosis, but the truth was that she had a real soft spot for Rufus, and it hurt to see him in pain and suffering. Hearing Delano say she was giving Mr. Brixton the best possible options somehow eased the stress she was under.

"Thanks," she said, completely forgetting her determination to keep her distance and touching his arm as she passed. A shock of warm electricity rushed into her hand, and she couldn't help noticing the firm muscles that bunched beneath his flesh. "I'll be back as soon as possible."

And she found herself absently rubbing her thumb and fingers together as she went back toward reception, trying to stop them tingling in reaction to the sensation of his skin beneath hers.

Delano released a rushed breath as the door closed behind Mellie, and looked down at the spot where she'd touched him. There was no mistaking the heat lingering on his arm, and the goose bumps that her light caress had caused to flare out across his back. But he pushed the sensation aside to consider another facet of Mellie's personality he thought he'd just figured out.

One of the things that had been emphasized by a professor at veterinary college was the fact that loving animals and wanting to help them all wasn't a secure enough basis to be a vet.

There's nothing wrong with having empathy for both animals and owners, she'd said. *But equally important for your own sanity is the understanding that you will not be able to cure or save every patient. Getting emotionally involved with all the animals you treat will eventually cause burnout.*

She'd gone on to explain that the suicide rate among animal welfare workers was one of the highest—on par with police officers and firefighters.

Watching Mellie examine Rufus, knowing she was both familiar with the animal and passionate about animal rescue, he'd found himself hyperfocused on her demeanor, trying to get a read on her emotional state. What he'd seen was a veterinarian who knew her job, was compassionate toward the patient and thoughtfully considerate to the owner's financial situation. Somehow she seemed to have found a balance between sentiment and the realities of her profession.

It made him feel much better about his decision not to ever come back to live on St. Eustace.

Just having to interact with the clients today had been emotionally exhausting. Many of them had known him when he was younger, and he swore a bunch only came into the clinic to be nosy. He'd examined animals that exhibited not one sign of disease, nor did they need any kind of preventative care. However, if the owners wanted to waste time and money just to get a look at Dr. Milo's errant son, who was he to complain?

The fuss would die down soon enough, when Delano left again.

In the meantime, he was beginning to think it would be politic to let Mellie know his plans didn't include taking over from his father. It seemed terribly unfair to him that she, who had put so much time and effort into the clinic, might be worrying about her future there.

He wasn't sure how to bring it up, though, without putting her back up.

Ten minutes later, the door swung open, revealing a sober Mellie.

"Mr. Brixton agreed that amputation is the best

option," Mellie said. "Although he's terribly upset at the idea."

"Rufus looks to be in good overall condition. I'm sure he'll do fine as a tripod, once he gets used to it."

Mellie nodded, looking at the chart where Delano had made some notes regarding the dog's condition while she was gone. "That's what I told him, but he's had Rufus since he was a puppy, so he's very attached." She flipped back a few pages of the chart, her eyebrows drawn together in concern. "Normally I'd have blood tests done to make sure he's in the best shape possible to withstand the stress of the operation, but he was in for his annual physical just two weeks ago, and everything was good."

A lucky happenstance, and another indication of the owner's commitment to his pet.

Mellie had pulled back up the X-rays, and was studying them intently.

"With the break where it is, I'll do a proximal femoral amputation," she muttered, talking more to herself than to him. "No need to make it more uncomfortable for him than necessary."

Delano had been thinking the same thing. Rather than take the leg off at the hip—coxofemoral disarticulation—which was necessary if the femur was damaged higher up, she was opting to leave a part of the bone intact. Not only was it a less invasive surgery, but because the thigh muscles would be sewn around the bone, the dog would be able to lie on that side more comfortably than if the entire leg was removed.

"Is Cecil back?" he asked, knowing Mellie usually had the surgical tech assist in delicate operations.

"No. He broke a tooth earlier and went to the dentist. He's still there." The wrinkles between her eyebrows deepened for an instant, and then smoothed out. Her expression, when she turned his way, was determined. "I don't want to wait for him to get back. Let's get started on this. I'll have reception warn clients coming in that there'll be a delay, and when Cecil gets back he can take over."

Glad not to have to face any more scrutiny from nosy patients just yet, Delano hastily agreed.

"While you're talking to Jackie, I'll get Rufus shaved."

And although the smile she sent his way was a little thin, it still gave him a warm sense of satisfaction.

Maybe there was hope for them to develop an easy working relationship, after all.

CHAPTER FIVE

MELLIE CAME BACK so quickly Delano was still using the shears to clip the hair on Rufus's leg prior to shaving down to the skin with a disposable razor. Bustling across the room, she looked over the instrument tray, then went to unlock the cupboard where the medicines were kept. Selecting the anesthesia, antibiotics and pain medications she'd be administering to Rufus prior to the start of the amputation, she took them over to the operating table.

There was a kind of controlled efficiency to her movements that Delano appreciated. She knew what she was about, and he could almost see the wheels turning in her head as she went over the operation in her head. And she knew how she liked everything arranged; Mellie had a system for organizing all the accoutrements necessary for the surgery ahead.

Going to the other side of the room, where the recovery cages were, she turned on the radio. Whoever had used it before had left it on the AM station, and the news blared out.

"...word from the head of the Trinidadian Racing Commission is that the Santa Rosa racetrack will reopen—"

Mellie hit a button, cutting the announcer off in

midsentence and filling the room with an R & B tune instead.

After turning the volume down to a more reasonable level, she said, "If I hear one more thing about the Racing Commission in Trinidad today, I think I might scream. No doubt you feel the same way."

He looked up at her to see if she was being facetious, but there was nothing but rueful amusement in her expression.

"Why would you say that?" he asked.

Now it was her turn to send him a searching look.

"Because almost every patient owner I've seen today has asked me something about what's happening, as if I have the inside scoop. I'm sure it's been even worse for you."

"Actually, no," he replied, turning back to shaving the last bit of stubble from Rufus's leg. "A couple of people sort of danced around the topic, but no one actually asked outright."

"Huh." The sound was somewhere between amusement and annoyance. "I think that must be some kind of weird instance of good manners overcoming normal nosiness, because I got a comprehensive grilling from everyone. Give them a few days to get used to the idea of you being here, and I'm betting that will change."

Delano couldn't help snorting. "They can hold off forever, if they like." Curiosity got the better of him, and he had to ask, "What did they want to know?"

The Racing Commission had played its cards close to its chest, revealing a minimum of information through the media and naming no names. Speculation had run rampant through Trinidad the day before Delano left for St. Eustace, and he could only figure the same was happening here.

"If it was a doping issue, or a betting scandal. If you were involved, and that's why you're here."

"Outrageous, when they all know Dad's ill." But he couldn't really put much weight behind the words, since there was a certain ugly logic to the speculation. That knowledge made him sigh, and although he tried to suppress the sound, it snuck out.

"Honestly, I had the same thoughts," Mellie admitted without rancor, but Delano was sure there was both an accusation and question behind her words, as though she were feeling him out.

As good a time as any to set her straight.

Focusing his gaze on where he was plying his razor, rather than on Mellie's face, Delano said, "I'm not sure how much information the commission has released, so please don't repeat this." He waited until she agreed before continuing, "They've been investigating a race-fixing ring for over six months, and I was asked to keep my eyes and ears open. I heard about Dad's heart attack, applied for leave and was about to book my ticket when it all came to a head, and they asked me to delay my departure until after I'd given a statement."

"So that's why you didn't make it here until Friday." Her voice was carefully noncommittal.

"Yes." Finally finished with shaving Rufus's leg, he put the razor into the bowl of water next to him, and faced Mellie. "I didn't have anything to do with the problem, other than to have been working at the track at the time it was going on. My job there is secure, and I'll be going back to it when my leave is up. Believe me, I won't be lingering here once I know Dad is on the mend and completely out of danger."

She didn't reply right away, her gaze searching his, as though trying to glean whether he was telling the truth or not. But although the moment should have simply been one that could determine the way they worked together going forward, Delano found himself holding his breath. He didn't understand why it was so important that Mellie believe him, but it was.

Mellie was equally still, her eyes dilated so there was a ring—almost golden—around the dark centers. A shiver worked its way up Delano's back, and had to be ruthlessly suppressed.

When she abruptly turned away, he couldn't be sure whether he was relieved or disappointed, especially when all she said was, "Okay," and indicated she was ready to start the operation.

As they prepared for the amputation, Delano realized he was thinking more about the woman competently readying herself than about the dog on the operating table, and pulled himself out of his ruminations.

There'd be time later to go back over the conversation, and try to figure out exactly what he was feeling, although a part of him whispered that he didn't actually want to know.

While she was concentrating on Rufus's surgery, and keeping an eye on how Delano handled himself during the operation, there was no time to contemplate what he'd said. But it lingered in the back of Mellie's mind nonetheless, awaiting a chance to come forward and be picked over.

About halfway through the surgery Cecil came back and took over from Delano, which Mellie found both a relief and disappointment. He had been a calm, capable presence in the room, handling the instruments and any assistance she needed with no fuss or questions.

It was hard not to appreciate the way he let her get on with her work without offering suggestions or trying to take over. Whatever she asked of him, he did, without any hesitation.

But, Mellie thought to herself after the surgery was over and Rufus was recovering under Cecil's supervision, just because he was a good vet and surgical partner, didn't mean he was trustworthy.

She wanted to believe him, both for Dr. Milo's sake and her own, but had learned a long time ago to be realistic with how she viewed people, and what they were capable of.

Her mother had been the first source of this knowledge.

Even as a child, Mellie had known her mother was difficult—exacting and derisive when her standards weren't met. Muddling through childhood, adolescence and early adulthood, trying to be everything expected of her, even while her self-assurance was being undermined by constant criticism, had been bad enough. Discovering Mom had lied to destroy the relationship between Mellie and her father had created a rift that would never completely heal.

Mellie had been told her father was a bum and deadbeat while, in reality, he'd not only been paying child support, but also sending gifts and letters from St. Eustace to Chicago.

None of which Mellie had received.

Only as an adult had Mellie allowed curiosity about her father to get the better of her, and she'd reached out to him. It had felt like the right time in her life. She'd been about to graduate vet school and, having mostly lived apart from her mother for the last few years, was feeling more confident about her ability to deal with whatever she discovered.

When her father had burst into tears and admitted her mother had told him Mellie never wanted anything to do with him, she'd cried too, but with mingled joy and rage.

When confronted, her mother had had a complete meltdown, calling Mellie ungrateful and a lot of other even more hurtful names, before saying she didn't want to have anything more to do with her.

Over the years, Mellie had tried to keep the lines of communication open, but her mother was always cool, dismissive and on occasion downright mean. When Kyle had conned her, it hadn't even occurred to Mellie to ask her mother for help. Instead, she'd turned to her father, and had never regretted that decision.

It had led her to St. Eustace, and the happiest days of her life. The first place she'd felt completely at home and accepted.

As though knowing she was thinking about him, her phone rang, the distinctive tone telling her it was her father on the other end. Sitting at her desk, figuring no one could begrudge her a few minutes respite after surgery, she answered.

"Hi, Daddy. I was just thinking about you."

"Good thoughts, I hope?"

"Always," she replied, with a chuckle, awash with love for the one person in the world she could say she completely trusted. "Although, when you call me at work, I do worry about what's going on."

His laughter lifted her spirits and she leaned back, rocking the chair slightly.

"You know me too well," Dad said. "Actually, I was wondering if you could come by and take a look at Lawrie? He's favoring his left hind leg, and his fetlock feels hot."

"Oh, do you need me to come now?" Lawrie was

one of her father's polo ponies, and the apple of his eye. "We have a waiting room full of people."

"No. Tomorrow will be fine. We wrapped the leg, and he doesn't seem to be in too much distress."

"I'll come by in the morning, or get Delano to go." It would get the darn man out of the clinic for a while, which suited Mellie just fine. "If that works for you?"

"Sure. You know I'm up from six, so any time after that works." He paused for a moment, then continued, "It would be nice to see Delano again. It's been a very long time."

It was an opening she really wanted to take advantage of. Her curiosity about the relationship between Dr. Milo and his son had grown day by day, and her father was one of Milo's best friends. She didn't doubt he could give her important insight into the situation.

"Dad..." It felt so wrong to ask her father about the Logan family dynamic, but there was something brewing—like a storm on the horizon—and she needed to be equipped to deal with it. "What's the story between Dr. Milo and Delano?"

There was a long pause, as though her father was thinking about not answering, but then he sighed.

"You know how Iris died, right?"

"Yes." Delano's mother had drowned off Ludlow Beach, trying to save a little boy caught in a riptide. At least, that was the story Mellie had heard.

"It tore that family apart." Mellie could hear the

remembered pain in her father's voice. "Milo was devastated, of course, and retreated into himself. And Delano...well, he'd lost both his mother and his best friend."

The sudden pang of sympathy and understanding she felt made her breath catch in her throat. "Janice Gopaul's son was Delano's best friend?"

She knew Janice well, since the older woman was one of the volunteers that helped out with the shelter outreach programs and the spay and neuter clinics. Someone had mentioned the connection between Dr. Milo and Janice to Mellie and, although she'd never discussed it with either of them, the information had stuck in her mind.

It had been such a huge tragedy, even now, more than twenty years later, people still remembered and occasionally spoke about it.

"Everard Gopaul. Yes, he was. Overnight, the relationship between Milo and Delano changed, and I don't think it ever recovered."

"Do you think that would be enough to make Delano not want to stay here, even if he has the chance to take over the clinic? It was a long time ago."

"Mel, he left here after high school, and hardly looked back." As her father was talking, Mellie saw the door to the office start to open, and felt a wash of embarrassment when Delano stepped in. Their eyes met, and he gave her a crooked smile, but she averted her gaze, hoping he wouldn't realize she was talking about him. Thank goodness her father had a relatively soft voice! "I can only think of two times that he's been back here—once for his grandfather's funeral, the other for one of his cousin's weddings. I don't see that antipathy toward the island changing anytime soon."

Although Delano had walked over to the other desk and seemed to be looking for something, Mellie wondered if he'd figured out that he was the topic of discussion. Not waiting to see if her father had anything to add, Mellie quickly said, "Okay, Daddy. Thanks, but I have to go back to work. I'll let you know who's coming tomorrow. Love you."

"Love you too, Mellie-Mel."

As she hung up, Delano turned to face her, and his eyebrows quirked.

"That was your father? How is Mr. Charlie?"

"He's good," she replied, tamping down the flustered sensation making her face feel too warm. "One of his polo ponies needs looking at, though. Do you think you could manage to get up to the farm and examine him tomorrow morning?"

"Sure. He's in the same place, isn't he?"

"Yes. Crispin Farm, in the valley just over the Rio Vida bridge."

"I remember it well. What time is he expecting me?"

"He's up at the barns from six in the morning, so any time after that will work for him," she replied, getting to her feet, and sliding out from around the desk. "I better get back to work. I saw how many patients we still have to see."

"I can manage awhile longer, if you need a break. That was a long operation, and did you even have lunch before we started?"

The expression on his face made another wave of warmth rush through her. It wasn't born from shame, though, but from the sensation that he really cared.

Then she scoffed silently at her gullibility. Hadn't she learned not to be taken in by charm and the illusion of concern?

Yet, she couldn't bring herself to snap at him. Suddenly the man she'd been thinking of as some kind of sneaking charlatan had taken on a more complex and sympathetic aura. So she just shook her head as she reached for the doorknob, and said, "It's all good. Let's get going."

But she could have sworn his gaze was boring into her back as she walked away.

CHAPTER SIX

BY THE END OF the day, Mellie was satisfied with Rufus's progress, although the dog seemed listless and a little down.

"Sorry, fella," she told him, after the clinic had closed and she was doing her last rounds. Rather than taking him out of the cage, she'd sat down on the ground next to it to examine him. Seeing the sadness in his eyes, she stayed a little longer after checking his drain and incision site, just to keep him company. "I know you're not feeling your best, and probably would prefer to be home, but we're taking good care of you."

"He doesn't seem too reassured."

The sound of Delano's voice, low and mellow, startled her, and Mellie's head jerked up as she turned to look at him.

"He's still a bit groggy, and unsure because it's so strange," she mumbled, stroking the dog's head. She still felt weird about what had happened earlier, and it made her revert to her prior stiffness. "I'm sure he'll be okay once he settles in."

Delano moved closer, then sat down next to her so he could also pet the mongrel.

"I always feel bad about leaving the animals overnight in the hospital," he admitted. "Even though I'm pretty sure they'll be okay, there's a part of me that worries anyway."

"I know," she agreed. It was difficult to strike the balance between professionalism and very genuine concern, and sometimes people took her empathy toward the animals as a type of weakness. Yet, she didn't hesitate to confide in Delano. "They can't articulate it the way we can, but I know they fret at being left in a strange place, especially when they're in pain."

"That's true, but he won't be with us for long."

"Hopefully," she replied, determined to break the intimacy of their conversation and move away from his too-close proximity.

What was it about him that drew her in against her will, and rendered her weak in the knees?

No matter what it was, she told herself sternly, she refused to give in to it. And staying here in the quiet of the after-hours clinic, so close that she could feel the warmth from his skin and smell the remnants of his cologne, was a bad idea.

As she rose to her feet, Delano stroked behind Rufus's ear again, and the dog gave him such a sad look he kept doing it.

Looking up at her, he asked, "Are you coming to obedience class tonight?"

She'd been thinking about it, wanting to see Delano take Baldur through his paces. No, actually what she'd fantasized about was seeing Delano in a tracksuit or shorts, running around. The Dobe was beautiful, but to Mellie his owner was even more so.

It would be yummy to see all those muscles in motion. Just the thought sent a trickle of desire along her veins.

For that very reason, she replied, "I don't think so. I need to get home and help Johnny Luck with the animals, and it would be nice to have a quiet evening at home. The last week has been stressful and tiring."

"Understandable," he replied.

He was still sitting on the floor and tilted his head back to look at her. It gave Mellie a new and strangely tantalizing view of his face, and her breath hitched in her chest as her gaze landed and clung to his lips.

Delano had a mouth made for kissing—truly he did. It was full-lipped, but eminently masculine at the same time, with a natural upturn at the corners that took it from attractive into the "sinful" category.

The temptation to bend and put her mouth on his was almost overwhelming, and when the tip of his tongue slipped out to dampen his lower lip, a shudder of desire heated Mellie's skin.

No. No. No.

This wouldn't do at all!

She spun on her heel and, in her haste, wobbled. Delano grabbed her leg, high up on her thigh, apparently trying to stabilize her balance. But what he did, instead, was make her gasp at the strength of his grip and the warmth of his palm evident through her scrubs.

"You okay there?"

His voice sounded even deeper than before, and the tone sent another shiver down her spine. Galvanized into action by the unwanted attraction weakening her knees, Mellie stepped carefully away and swallowed to make sure her voice wouldn't croak.

"Yes." Intent on sounding unmoved, it came out cold, as sharp as ice. "I'm fine."

Hearing the gate to the kennel close, she risked a glance over her shoulder. He'd shot the bolt home and, as she watched, rose to his feet with fluid grace, giving her a fine view of his glutes and thigh muscles at work.

Before he could catch her staring, Mellie looked down at the chart on the table in front of her, although she couldn't for the life of her remember which animal's it was.

"Well, I'm going to head out so I can get ready for class."

He sounded normal again, making Mellie wonder if she'd imagined the change in his tone before.

"Okay," she replied, assiduously avoiding looking his way and keeping her voice level. "See you tomorrow."

"Night."

She stayed where she was, not moving a muscle until she heard him call for Baldur and exit through the rear door of the clinic. In fact, she didn't relax until the sound of his car engine faded into the distance.

Then the air left her lungs with a *whoosh*, and she put her elbows on the table and her head in her hands.

What on earth was she doing? The very last thing she needed or wanted was to be drooling over Delano Logan. Sure, her instinctive distrust for him and his motivations had waned, but if she were smart, she'd hang on to at least some of her suspiciousness.

He claimed to be in the clear with the Racing Commission, and determined to go back to Trinidad as soon as he possibly could, but there was a part of her that still couldn't bring itself to believe him.

Maybe it was because she'd found her place—and her true, authentic self—here on St. Eustace, and found it impossible to fathom why anyone else wouldn't feel the same.

Her life was busy, and fulfilling, but she also had friends and a social life. She worked hard, but there was the opportunity to play just as hard, whenever she wanted. Since arriving here, the stress of trying to be what others expected her to be had finally fallen away, and she could chart her own course.

Or had felt as though she could, until Delano had turned up.

As attracted to him as she was, she couldn't lose sight of the fact he had the power to completely undo almost everything she'd built.

Including, she acknowledged to herself, her hard-won self-esteem. She was honest enough to admit she wanted to sleep with him, but the thought of him turning out to be unworthy of her trust was a barrier she'd find hard to overcome.

The old lesson—that caring for and even loving someone didn't mean they had your best interests at heart, or wouldn't lie for their own gains—was ingrained on her psyche. Carved there by her mother, and reinforced by Kyle. And unless she could trust Delano, and be assured her emotions wouldn't be involved, so when he left she wouldn't be devastated, he was definitely off-limits!

However difficult it might be, she had to revert to her previous manner of treating him: putting aside all sympathy, quashing any overtures of friendship, maintaining her distance.

She could do that, couldn't she?

But there was no great confidence behind her determination, and Mellie knew it.

The obedience class ended at eight that evening, and Delano thankfully waved goodbye to the last participant before heading to the car with Baldur heeling at his side.

The class had been a bit of a shambles. Along with the eight or so people his father had told him to expect, there'd been another five newcomers. Those five, like some of the clients at the clinic, seemed to be there strictly out of curiosity, since the dogs were completely uncontrollable and the handlers had no idea what they were doing.

At least he'd had the satisfaction of getting them started on the road to having well-trained dogs, if the novelty didn't wear off before they got to that point.

Restless, and unwilling to go home right away, Delano decided to pick up some takeout and swing by the clinic to check on Rufus and keep him company for a while. The dog had shown signs of depression—not unusual after surgery and being away from home—and Delano had made a point to visit him as often as possible throughout the day. Just like with humans, an animal's ability to heal, and do so quickly, very often was affected by their mood.

Driving along through the downtown area, he felt a wave of nostalgia at the small food shops and vendors lining the road. The fare on offer in Port Michael reflected the diversity of the St. Eustace population—doubles and stuffed roti jostled for space alongside "pan" chicken, roasted corn and slabs of salted fish. Other vendors offered soups and stews, such as pepper pot, and the children gravitated to the crushed ice covered with syrup, served in little plastic bags, or a variety of sweet baked goods.

No matter what you had a hankering for, you could find it, or something similar, along Garvey Road.

Everard and he used to spend most of the week-ends and school holidays riding their bicycles all over Port Michael, and Delano remembered them heading here at the end of the day. By then, having visited the beach or the fishing village at the edge of the city, or whatever other mischief they'd gotten up to, they'd be starving. The vendors knew when they had money they'd spend it all on the street food, but when they were broke Everard, with his careless charm, would often get something for free.

Everard.

As was usually the case when his thoughts turned to his childhood best friend, his first instinct was to push all memories aside. It was what he'd done for over twenty years, since just thinking his name once more brought that agonizing rush of shame, guilt and loss. That had worked in Trinidad, but suddenly felt impossible here.

Around every corner there was something to remind him of Everard.

And Mum.

No.

He wasn't going down that road. Not tonight. Not any other night if he had his way.

Their deaths were far, far in the past, and he refused to allow them to drag him back down into the dark place he'd lived in for years after they'd happened.

Stopping the car next to a chicken stand, he ordered a meal, and determinedly engaged the vendor in chatter while he waited. As he took the foil package from the vendor and thanked him, he saw Baldur's nose go up in the air.

"Oh, no, my friend," Delano told the dog. "You already had your dinner earlier. This is all mine."

Not that Baldur would expect to get any, since Delano didn't allow his animals to eat human food. But the dog was a master of the begging eyes and seemed to always live in hope that his doleful expression would finally bear fruit.

As he drove toward the clinic, Delano mused on his conversations with Mellie earlier in the day, and then again that evening.

He hoped he'd made it plain to her that she had nothing to fear from him, when it came to her place at the clinic. That he had no intention of staying and usurping her position.

It wasn't hard to understand why she worried. Dad had made oblique references to retirement, as though he was sounding Delano out, while Aunt Eddie had been far more direct.

"Your father would be so happy to see his life's work continue on," she'd said. "Especially if you were a part of that."

"The clinic is in good hands with Mellie," he'd retorted. "And Dad hasn't said he's ready to retire just yet."

He'd been hoping she wouldn't pursue the conversation but, of course, Aunt Eddie wouldn't be deterred until she'd had her full say.

"He might not have said it outright, but he is.

And Mellie is completely competent," she agreed readily. "But there's work enough for two."

It made him feel hemmed in and put on the spot. All he wanted was to get back to Port of Spain and away from the barrage of memories.

At least, that's what he had to keep telling himself.

There was something about Mellie that often made him forget that St. Eustace wasn't somewhere he wanted to be.

The thread of attraction he felt toward her, which no matter how hard he tried wouldn't be ignored, overshadowed all else. Even when she was coolly sassing him or giving him the side-eye, he was totally aware of her as a woman...her movements, scent, expressions.

More than once he'd found himself fixated on her lips, the urge to test their softness with his, to taste them, almost overwhelming. Like this evening, when it had felt like an electric current was flowing through the air around them, and it had taken every ounce of willpower he had not to get up and take her into his arms.

Kiss her senseless. Or until he, himself, was senseless, and all his pain, sorrow and guilt fell away.

Yet, he knew himself well. Well enough to admit there was a permanent emotional barrier between him and other people. One he'd carefully built up over the years, and no longer thought could be breached. He'd tried honestly during his marriage to let his wife into his heart, but Stella had known he wasn't all in. She'd said as much, during the trainwreck days as it fell completely apart.

You don't have the capacity to love, Delano. Her words had cut through him, even as he'd had to acknowledge their truth. *You have no heart. You don't care about anyone.*

Realistically, her indictment had made him feel horrible and less than he should be, but he made no effort to change.

Getting too close to others opened yourself up to devastation, and he'd had more than enough of that in his life as it was. Yet, his father's health scare forced him to admit he wasn't fully immune to connections of the heart. It had scared him into realizing how much his father meant to him, even if Milo didn't feel quite the same way.

Turning into the clinic, he was surprised to see lights on in the hospital area, and Mellie's car parked out back. Immediately his heart started pounding in anticipation, and he almost drove back out of the parking lot. Still, although he hesitated for a long moment before turning off the ignition, he knew he would be going inside anyway.

CHAPTER SEVEN

AFTER GETTING HIMSELF and Baldur out of the vehicle, Delano grabbed his dinner and let himself into the clinic via the side door, which led right into the hospital.

Mellie had turned on only one light in the other room, leaving the hospital in low, golden light, and was sitting on the floor beside Rufus's cage, her little mutt, Sheba, lying beside her. Sheba's whip tail beat a tattoo of greeting on the floor, while Mellie gave him a bland stare, without a hint of welcome. The change from earlier, when there'd seemed to be a distinct thawing of her attitude toward him, took him aback and raised his hackles.

"What are you doing here?" she asked, in that cool, distant voice that so irritated him.

He smiled, or tried to, using the baring of his teeth to mask the sudden flood of annoyance.

"The same thing you are, I suspect," he replied, stopping himself from calling Baldur back to his side when the traitorous canine headed straight for Mellie, getting in her face for pets. "We came to keep Rufus company a little."

She glanced at Rufus, who was looking back and forth between them from beneath the edge of the cone he was wearing to stop him licking his wound. Delano looked at the dog too, noticing that his eyes seemed brighter, but his head was low and his tail didn't move.

"He has been a bit down," Mellie conceded. "He misses his owner."

Pulling a stool up to the nearest counter, Delano unwrapped his chicken from its foil envelope, said, "Well, he has as much company as he can get right now. Maybe having Baldur and Sheba here will help too."

The sound she made was no doubt supposed to be some kind of agreement, but to Delano it immediately brought other, more erotic situations to mind.

He cleared his throat, suddenly glad he was on the opposite side of the table, where she wouldn't be able to notice his physical reaction. And how ridiculous that response was, when taken in the context of Mellie reverting to her cool, distancing persona. It was as though the accord they'd achieved earlier had never happened, or had been a figment of his imagination.

"How did obedience class go?"

Delano chuckled around a mouthful of food, then swallowed.

"It was a mess. There were five people there who hadn't a clue. One of the dogs even tangled me in their lead and tripped me. I went down like a felled tree. Never been more embarrassed in my life."

Mellie's gurgle of amusement lightened the atmosphere, and lifted his spirits. In between bites of his dinner, he regaled her with all the mishaps and comedic faux pas of the evening, just happy to hear her laughter ringing through the air.

Finished with his meal, he wadded up the foil and, ignoring Baldur's baleful stare, tossed the refuse into the garbage bin. Then he hesitated for a moment, torn.

Mellie was still sitting in front of the cage, Sheba pressed close to her side, the little mongrel's head on her lap. It would be politic to go back and sit on the stool where he'd been before, but Delano felt drawn to Mellie's side, and gave in to the impulse to get closer to her.

When he stepped over to where she sat, Mellie silently shuffled over to allow him room to sit on her other side. Delano settled onto the concrete, trying to make himself as small as possible so as not to crowd her, but it was impossible for their bodies not to touch in the confined space.

Especially when Baldur came and leaned against Delano, his sturdy weight pressing his master into even closer proximity to Mellie. Now there was no ignoring the warmth emanating from her skin, and the soft, sweet scent filling his nostrils. Mellie shifted, not away, though, but just in place so her arm rubbed against his, leaving behind a trail of fire. Delano's body tightened; a hot shiver started at the base of his spine and ran up to his nape, leaving goose bumps in its wake.

"Baldur, down." His voice was gruff, the sudden rush of desire making him harsher than he meant to be, and he gave the dog a little nudge with his elbow. Then, getting himself back under control, he said to Mellie, "Sorry about that. He weighs a ton."

"No worries," she replied, but she shifted farther over, as though to give him additional room, lessening his discomfort.

They were quiet for a moment and, as he reached out to stroke Rufus, Delano wrestled his desire into submission.

It had been a while since he'd been attracted to a woman as strongly as he was to Mellie, but he knew this was someone he had to tread gently with. Not only was she his father's employer and friend, but he realized he genuinely liked her—cared about her well-being. She was, in effect, the last woman he would want to hurt in any way.

Best and far easier for all involved to keep their relationship friendly, even if he couldn't maintain the type of distance he normally found easy enough to preserve between him and others.

In the dim golden light, Delano gradually relaxed and turned his thoughts to something he'd wondered about for a while, but had never pursued.

"Can I ask you something?"

Mellie shrugged, smiling slightly.

"Sure."

"How come we never knew each other when we were kids? I mean, our fathers are good friends. Even though I know you lived abroad, I would have thought you'd spend some time here. Summers, or Christmas vacation."

Her sudden stillness made him wonder if he'd strayed into an area of her life she'd rather not discuss, and it was on the tip of his tongue to retract the question. But then she drew in a deep breath and released it on a sigh.

"I didn't get to know my dad until I was in my late twenties, so I never had the chance to visit when I was young."

The shock of that made his mouth dry, and although he wondered how that could have been, all he said was, "I'm sorry."

She shook her shoulders, as though sloughing something off. "Don't be. It turned out all right." Sending him a searching glance over her shoulder, she continued, "I'm surprised you didn't know that already." Then she chuckled, and said, "Actually, I'm not. Dr. Milo never gossips about anything."

"He despises gossip," Delano agreed.

"Do you know how many times I've come to tell him something or other, and he's said, 'I already know'? Drives me nuts."

He couldn't help grinning. "You're not the first woman to complain about that. Aunt Eddie does too, and my mother used to, as well. Mum would fuss at him because people told him all kinds of things, but he never passed any of it on. Mum said it was like being married to a priest who couldn't divulge what he'd heard in confession."

Mellie laughed so hard, she snorted, and the vibrations of her amusement transferred through where their legs rested against each other. "That's the perfect description."

While he laughed with her, it took Delano a moment to realize he'd spoken about his mother without feeling anything but love and amusement. Usually he pushed thoughts of her aside to avoid the inevitable sorrow and guilt. But somehow, with Mellie, he could bring out a happy, funny memory, and think of Mum with laughter and fond appreciation for her witty turns of phrase.

Then Mellie's amusement faded and she nibbled on her bottom lip, regarding him through eyes narrowed by a little frown.

"I'm going to say something, and I hope you'll take it in the spirit meant, because I'm not trying to hurt you, or put you on a guilt trip."

Delano stiffened, and the glow of contentment he'd felt just seconds before evaporated.

"Okay," he responded, stretching the word out, wondering where this conversation was going and bracing himself for whatever she came up with.

"Through no fault of his own, Daddy and I were estranged," she started, speaking slowly, as though picking her words with care. "Once we got back in touch and developed a relationship, it was the best thing that ever happened to me. Now my only regret is that we missed all those years of knowing each other."

She was trying to sound factual, but Delano thought he heard an undercurrent of residual pain in her voice. Mellie's gaze was firmly focused on his, and her sincerity was unmistakable when she continued to speak. Yet, his muscles tightened, knowing she was probably about to say something he didn't want to hear.

"Your father is a good man. He's decent and kind and logical. You seem to take after him in that respect, as far as I can see. Whatever happened between you to cause a rift, don't you think it's time to mend it? Even if you're determined to go back to Trinidad, wouldn't it be better to do that with both of you knowing your relationship is solid?"

And the pain her words caused him made him retreat, unwilling to face it or the woman gazing at him with both compassion and determination.

As Mellie spoke, she'd seen Delano's expression change, grow closed and distant, but she knew if she hadn't spoken up, she'd regret it later. Dr. Milo was her mentor and friend, and whether Delano realized it or not, their fractured relationship upset the older man intensely.

Just as the silence between them was becoming uncomfortable, Delano stirred, as though he'd been far away, and the corners of his mouth quirked upward. Not into a smile, exactly, but a facsimile of one—forced and unnatural.

"I'm not sure there's anything I can do about my relationship with Dad, but I'll take what you said under advisement. After all, you know him better at this stage than I do."

It was on the tip of her tongue to ask him whose

fault that was, but although his expression was carefully neutral, Mellie was sure there was veiled pain behind his dark eyes.

She knew better than most people just how heartbreaking estrangement from a parent could be. And while she still had her father to make the situation with her mother a little easier, Delano's mother had been gone for a long time.

No matter how close he might be with his aunt Eddie, there really was no compensating for a mother's love.

Delano looked down to where his hand slowly resumed stroking behind Rufus's ear, and Baldur sidled closer, resting his head on his owner's lap, as though in sympathy.

"I don't know how to make things better with Dad," he said quietly, as though the words were being drawn out of him unconsciously. As if he were talking more to himself than to her. "He won't discuss the past, and I…" For a moment she thought he wouldn't continue, but then he sighed, and said, "And I can't seem to put it all behind me. There were things that happened—that were said…"

His voice faded, leaving Mellie with an insistent sense of empathetic sadness. Without thought, she put an arm around his shoulders and gave him a little squeeze.

"I hear you," she said. "But sometimes even when we can't get at the answers, we really do need to move forward from where we are. Not leave the past behind us, necessarily, but accept we might never know everything we want to, and admit the present and future might just be more important."

He turned his head, so they were face-to-face, and his gaze sought and captured hers.

"Is that what you did—when you came here? After you found your father again?"

He was so close his breath touched her lips, and the intimacy of the moment had warmth blooming in her chest. She wanted—oh-so badly—to kiss him, but the conversation was too serious to abandon.

"It was more than just rediscovering Dad that brought me here. But yes, I definitely had to remind myself I wasn't the sum total of my family's secrets and my own stupid mistakes so as to move forward. And thrive."

His eyebrows rose, but she could no longer see the expression in his eyes, because his lids had fallen to half-mast. Something about the way he looked had her heart racing, and released a plethora of butterflies into her stomach.

"Secrets and mistakes, eh?" He was almost whispering, his voice rumbling and causing an answering echo in her torso. "You tell me yours, and I'll tell you mine…"

"Maybe." She found herself whispering too, and the distance between their mouths was suddenly too far. Or too close. Her addled brain couldn't decide which, stuck on wondering how he would taste, and whether he would be as good a kisser as she thought. "One day. Not tonight."

These moments were too sweet to disrupt with the ugliness of the world outside.

"No," he agreed, his gaze dropping to her lips. "Not tonight."

Was it an invitation? Mellie didn't know, but she was suddenly willing to take a chance and find out. Every inch of her flesh tingled with anticipation, and her heart was set to hammer its way out of her chest.

If she didn't kiss Delano, she thought she might spontaneously combust.

As she began to tilt her head toward his, she hesitated, wondering if she should ask, but it was a moot point since he met her halfway and their lips touched. Softly at first, testing and molding, learning the contours of each other's mouth, breathing each other in with inhalations that grew increasingly rushed.

When the tip of his tongue swept her lower lip, Mellie shuddered, shocked by the intensity of her reaction, which swept out from her belly to heat every inch of her being.

She was insensate to everything but Delano—his scent and warmth, the hardness of his shoulders beneath her arm, the tenderness of his hand cupping her cheek, angling her perfectly for his kiss.

They both jumped, startled, when Sheba let out a sudden volley of barks then took off across the room and out the door toward reception. Baldur, although holding his position beside Delano, added his own deep warning.

Yet, even when someone knocked loudly on the front door, neither Mellie nor Delano moved, their gazes once more meshing, questioning. Was he trying to come to terms with what had just happened, the way she was?

"I should see who that is," she said, shocked by the rawness in her throat, which rendered her voice whiskey-rough.

"Yeah," he agreed, but his hand, which was now on the side of her throat, didn't drop away.

For some reason, that made her huff with a little burst of amusement, and her heart did a strange dip when his lips curled into a smile.

It was Sheba's increasingly frantic barking that had her tearing her gaze away from his and somehow getting to her feet. Her legs felt shaky and, as she followed Sheba into the reception area, she touched the tip of her tongue to her lower lip, searching for one last taste of Delano.

Switching on the light outside the front door of the clinic so she could see who was outside, hyper-aware of Delano coming into the room, she pushed aside the blinds and looked out.

"Who is it?" he asked, standing way too close for comfort.

It made her want to ignore the person outside, and drag Delano back into their office and ravish him.

For the sake of her sanity, she shifted away, putting a modicum of distance between them.

"A taxi driver I know," she replied, turning the

lock. Pulling open the door, she tried to smile at the diminutive gentleman standing on the doorstep and holding a cardboard box. "Hi, Mr. Jolly. What's going on?"

"I was coming down Pepper Hill, Dr. Mellie, and a woman flag me down and ask me if I coming to town and if I can bring you this." From the meows coming from the box, Mellie already had a good idea of the contents even before Mr. Jolly continued, "She say the mama puss disappear yesterday, and she don't see her come back, so she 'fraid the little one's going dead without them mother. If the lights wasn't on here, I'd have take them up to your house."

More kittens, when she'd just found homes for the six she'd bottle-raised over last month! But, of course, there was no way she could or would refuse.

Taking the box from Mr. Jolly, she said, "Okay, but next time you're going back through Pepper Hill, if you see that woman tell her if the mother cat comes back, she should contact me about getting her spayed so she won't have any more kittens."

"I will." The taxi driver smiled, gesturing over his shoulder. "She send you some jelly coconuts too, Dr. Mellie, for your trouble."

"I'll get them," Delano offered, slipping by her to follow Mr. Jolly to the car, leaving a heated spot on her arm where he'd brushed against it.

Mellie told herself to take the kittens back into the hospital yet she didn't move. Instead, she watched Delano walk alongside Mr. Jolly to the trunk of the car. Delano had a confident, sexy stride that commanded her attention.

How much simpler all this would be if she wasn't so intensely attracted to him. And now that she knew he was interested in her too, everything was even more complicated. She was mentally kicking herself for giving in to her desire.

What should she do now? Tell him it was a mistake? Pretend it didn't happen?

As Delano laughed at something Mr. Jolly said, Mellie's heart did a flip and heat flamed up from her belly into her face at the rich, decadent sound.

Maybe he could pretend that kiss was a figment of their imagination, but Mellie knew she wouldn't be able to.

Thankfully, just then Sheba stood up on her hind legs, nose snuffling at the bottom of the box, her tail wagging a mile a minute. It was just the distraction Mellie needed to stop mooning over the most handsome, fascinating and utterly frustrating man she'd ever met.

Slowly making her way to the hospital, Sheba prancing and jigging around her as she went, Mellie was still thinking about their prior conversation and its aftermath.

Delano came back inside and closed the front door, and Mellie heard the click of Baldur's nails on the tile along the corridor as she was opening the box.

"How many kittens?" Delano stood on the other side of the table and leaned to peer into the box.

"Looks like three," she replied, glad he seemed determined not to mention what had happened before, at least for a while. Reaching in, she pulled out the first kitten by its scruff.

"A ginger." Delano touched the tiny body, stroking down its back. "About four weeks old, do you think?"

"Yes, and that's such a relief to me," she said, trying to sound normal, although with the way her heart was pounding, she wasn't sure what that even meant anymore. Replacing the kitten in the box, she took out a fluffy gray one. "I just weaned and rehomed a litter of six and wasn't looking forward to having to bottle-feed another."

Delano nodded, bringing the smallest of the kittens out of the box, a little black ball of fur that gave an almost soundless hiss, which made Delano chuckle.

"Okay, tough guy," he said, juggling the squirming kitten. "I've got you, whether you like it or not."

"Can you confirm it's a guy and not a girl?" she asked. She'd had a look at both the ginger and the gray, and thought they were female, but the gender of kittens of this age was notoriously difficult to determine.

He laughed, whether at her question or the fact that the kitten was trying to run up his shirt, she wasn't sure.

"As confidently as anyone could be at this point," he replied, not putting the kitten back into the box with its siblings, but cradling it between his palms. "What are you going to name them?"

Tearing her gaze away from his hands, she stared blankly down into the box.

"I usually try to do linked names," she replied, her brain refusing to give his question its full attention. It was too busy wondering what it would feel like having those hands on her body. "It makes it easier to keep them all straight. The last ones were *Star Trek TNG* themed—Troi, Wesley, Riker, Worf, Jean-Luc, Beverly. I'm drawing a blank on these."

"How about going really retro?" he asked, actually bringing the kitten up to his face and snuggling it, making Mellie's heart melt. "Ginger, Mary Ann and Gilligan, for this dude?"

"I like that," she said, glad he'd come up with something since her brain was still stuck on their kiss. And the way he was cuddling the little black kitten, which was happily curled up in his hand, wasn't helping.

She wanted to be embraced like that!

Snap out of it, Mellie!

Hadn't she just been thinking how much more complicated life would be if she slept with Delano?

What she needed to do, right now, was make as graceful an exit as she could, and hopefully he'd get the hint and not mention what had happened before.

"I have to get these babies home," she said, making her voice brisk and businesslike. The little black kitten was fast asleep against Delano's chest, and

Mellie almost couldn't stand the cuteness. "I'll see you tomorrow."

"Yes," he replied, in a voice that sounded not one whit upset. He gently lowered the kitten into the box, and closed the flaps, while sending Mellie a little smile. "I'll see you in the morning."

And while she was walking to the car, Mellie was cursing herself for swinging wildly between elation at their sudden intimacy and disappointment at the easy way he'd let her leave.

CHAPTER EIGHT

SEVEN THIRTY THE next morning found Delano crossing the Rio Vida, on his way back from Charlie Roscoe's farm.

The visit had gone better than he'd expected. Mr. Charlie—as Delano had called him since he was a child—was the same forthright man he'd always been, but unlike almost everyone else on the island didn't pry into the younger man's business. He'd been welcoming and chatty, and the only sort of touchy moment was when he'd asked how Delano liked working with Mellie.

Thankfully, Delano was bending over looking at Lawrie's leg when he asked.

"She's a really good vet," he replied, glad that Mr. Charlie couldn't see his face. "Great with patients and their owners too."

And a fantastic kisser!

But Mr. Charlie didn't seem to notice anything strange in what he'd said, and replied, "She is, isn't she? I keep telling her to just concentrate on the veterinarian side of things, and not bother with all this animal rescue business, but she won't listen."

Without thinking, Delano said, "She's passionate about rescuing. It seems to make her happy."

Mr. Charlie sighed. "Oh, I know it, and I wouldn't

do anything to get in her way. I just worry about her emotional health. Rescuers have to have thick skins, and yet the majority—like Mellie—don't."

"She probably has a thicker skin than most," he replied, wondering why he felt as though he had to defend her to her father. "Being a vet isn't for bleeding hearts."

"True." There was a thoughtful tone to Mr. Charlie's voice. "I never really thought about it that way."

They'd left the conversation there, much to Delano's relief.

He'd already spent most of the previous night tossing and turning, thoughts of Mellie making him alternatively confused and aroused. Just the fact that he'd spoken to her about both his parents—especially his mother—without hesitation and without much pain had been surprising enough. But then add that kiss on to it, and he'd been knocked completely for a loop.

The damned woman had well and truly gotten under his skin, and he wasn't sure what to do about it.

He'd done his best to reassure her his plans didn't include staying in St. Eustace. He'd be a fool not to realize his father's heart attack, coupled with Delano's arrival had created an aura of uncertainty regarding the future of the clinic.

And who knew what Dad had said or intimated to Mellie.

Their kiss the night before had been amazing. He'd wanted more and more of her, but, at the same time, it had scared him silly. It had felt so right, so important, he couldn't help wondering if Mellie had felt the same way.

If, in her mind, it had somehow negated what he'd said about leaving.

Not that she struck him as the type of woman to build fantasies out of one kiss.

Maybe, a voice whispered, he was worried not because of what Mellie felt about it but because of how *he* felt.

It wouldn't hurt, though, to make sure they were on the same page—about the clinic, the kiss and the future. And doing it outside of work seemed like the best way.

All in all, it was far too easy to make the decision to see if she was still at home, and have an even franker conversation than they'd had prior.

So, telling himself the startling intimacy they'd shared the night before had nothing to do with his plan, he turned on to Bromfield Road, knowing her property was somewhere along it, not too far from town.

Bromfield Road cut through the hills from south to north and his hope to find Mellie's place before he got too far away from Port Michael came true sooner than he expected. Rounding a corner revealed a wide, flat valley sloping away to the right while on the left the land plateaued the way it sometimes did in the midst of the rolling hills. The land on the left was fully enclosed with a high chain-link fence and, standing on the driveway, hanging on to two ropes, one in either hand, was Mellie.

At the end of the ropes were a pair of goat kids that seemed determined to play tug-of-war with Mellie in the middle. Her arms were stretched out wide to either side, while the goats appeared to have dug their little hooves in, resisting with all their might whatever it was she was trying to get them to do.

But what caught and completely arrested Delano's attention was the mirth on Mellie's face.

She was laughing, head thrown back. Sheer, unfettered joy radiated from every line and curve of her body and face. At that moment, bathed in the subtle early morning light, she was almost more beautiful than he could bear.

And he wanted her beyond all reason.

Pulling his car onto the grass verge near her gate then turning off the ignition, he sat watching her a moment more before getting out. As he was about to close the door, one of the kids reared up on its hind legs and cocked its head to the side in a motion that anyone familiar with goats would instantly recognize. But as the little rascal tottered toward Mellie, it lost its balance and tumbled over, and Mellie's peals of laughter turned into howls.

Delano couldn't help laughing too at the ridiculous expression on the kid's face. It sprang back to its hooves and looked around, as though to check whether anyone else saw its embarrassing fall.

The snap of the car door closing attracted Mellie's attention and, on seeing him, her laughter intensified.

"Did you see that?" she gasped, trying to stem the hilarity and only partially succeeding. "These two crack me up."

"I did," Delano replied, his heart pounding like a hammer on an anvil. It was the sight of that grin, and the light visible in her eyes even from a distance that made him feel as though the earth had tilted, and he was about to fall off. "He's a real silly Billy, huh?"

He could have kicked himself for the corny joke, but Mellie went into another spate of giggles.

"Right? Frick and Frack never stop making me laugh." She cocked an eyebrow at him. "You coming in? The dogs are all locked away, so it's safe."

The property was encircled by a six-foot-high chain-link fence with an automatic gate, but there was also a pedestrian gate and Delano lifted the latch and pushed it open. "Frick and Frack?" he queried, as he closed and locked the gate behind him. "Where'd you get those names?"

"Originally these two jokers were Harry and Ron, but they get into so much trouble, and are so hilarious, I renamed them. Frick and Frack are what my dad calls any mischievous pair of people, so it seemed to fit. I think they were comedic skaters, way back when. At least, that's what he said."

"Suits them, then," he said, smiling back at her, hoping he didn't look as goofy as he felt. "Although the original names would be just as apt."

She nodded in agreement.

As though his presence inhibited the kids, they'd

scampered over to Mellie and stood, one on either side and just behind her legs, peering around at Delano.

"What brings you here so early?" Mellie asked, shortening the ropes and starting to walk toward a nearby pen. "Did you need directions to Dad's farm?"

"No." He fell in beside her, as the goats trotted off ahead of them, clearly knowing where they were supposed to go. "I'm just coming back from there actually."

Mellie sent him a quick sideways look. "How's Lawrie?"

"He'll be fine. I put on a poultice and suggested he be allowed to rest for at least a week."

"Dad must have been disappointed. He has a polo match this coming weekend, and Lawrie is his favorite mount."

"He seemed to take it all right." Delano stepped ahead of her to open the gate to the pen. "Your father strikes me as a man who'd prefer to ride his second string, rather than risk the well-being of his horses."

"He is," she agreed, shooting him an approving glance as she bent to remove the ropes from around the goats' necks. When she straightened, she asked, "So, with that settled, why are you here?"

He searched her face for a moment, but found only curiosity. Had she put their kiss out of her mind so quickly?

"Well, I thought we could have a conversation."

Now he was the one subjected to an interrogative look, and it was impossible to miss the flash of her eyes, or the light blush that rose to her cheeks.

So she did remember their kiss, and thought that was what he wanted to talk about.

Why that filled him with a ridiculous sense of masculine pride was something he didn't want to consider, and made an effort not to let it show in his expression.

But she sounded calm and collected when she pointed with her chin toward the cottage, and said, "Okay. Want some coffee?"

"Sure."

But then they stood there a moment longer, as though delaying what was to come. Watching the kids gambol and frisk toward a shaded area where a flock of chickens and a rather threadbare turkey were pecking the ground. There was also a lone sheep grazing along the fence line.

"Quite an array of animals you have here," he commented. "Somehow, I thought it would be mostly dogs and cats."

Mellie shrugged.

"I take any animal that needs help." She pointed at the sheep. "Dolly's owner had no idea what having sheep entailed. Thankfully, she only got the one, but when she decided to get rid of Dolly, I took her when it became clear no one else would.

"The chickens I raised myself, but Horatio, the turkey, was running wild and chasing people all over a neighborhood in Port Michael. No one seemed to know where he came from, but he can be quite ferocious, and I rescued him before he got run over or otherwise killed. I have a donkey and a pair of pigs too, at the back."

There was a note of defiance in her voice, as though she was continually having to justify the existence of the shelter. It made him sad, and a little angry too.

"I think what you're doing is admirable." That drew her attention, and he was sure he saw skepticism in her eyes, so he rushed to add, "I get so tired of seeing stray animals half-starved and neglected on the streets. If more people were like you—willing to try to do something about them—the world would be a better place."

She turned abruptly away, reaching for the latch on the gate before he realized what she was about to do.

"Come on," she said, her voice a little hoarse and almost brusque. "Let's get that coffee, and you can tell me what it is that brings you here at this time of morning."

Obviously she thought he was blowing smoke, but that wasn't what he was doing at all.

Hopefully her reaction to what he'd said wasn't an indication that she'd soured toward him again.

But he was reassured when, halfway across the space between the pen and her cottage, Mellie suddenly said, "I've found that most people want to do right by their animals. Some just don't know how, while others don't have the financial means to do it.

While we do see clear cases of cruelty, those are in the minority. Mostly it's injury and disease caused by a lack of knowledge or funds."

"So, what's the answer?" he asked, more to keep the conversation going than because he didn't have some ideas of his own.

"Education, primarily," she answered swiftly. "What a lot of people don't want to talk about is that not everyone is going to turn into a mushy animal owner who talks about their pets as 'fur babies.' For a lot of people, animals have particular purposes. If you can convince them those purposes are best served when the animals are taken care of, and give them the means and ability to do so, they'll be on board."

They'd climbed the three steps up to her veranda by then, and as she pushed open the door, a barrage of barks and furry creatures were waiting on the other side.

"Enough," Mellie said firmly to the dogs. "Outside, all of you."

The dogs obediently streamed out the door, along with one cat that stalked past Delano and gave him a snooty *who do you think you are?* look. Sheba paused to lick first Mellie then Delano, but also ran outside.

Once she shut the door, Mellie waved him through the living room to the back of the house, where he found himself in a kitchen just big enough for the appliances and a small table.

"Sit," Mellie said, walking over to the coffee

maker, which was burbling away. Delano took one of the wrought iron chairs, as directed, and shifted it so he could stretch out his legs.

"So, go on with what you were saying," he urged.

"Uh, where was I? Oh, yes. People who view animals as useful tools, rather than pets you bring into the house and coddle. There are certain myths around about what happens when people spay or neuter their animals—like they get lazy, and won't do the things they used to. People also do things like feed their dogs hot peppers, and keep them chained and unsocialized in the hopes of making them fiercer and better watchdogs. Those are some of the things we talk about, not just with the adults, but also through school programs arranged by the St. Eustace SPCA."

She gave a little chuckle as she took down a mug from the cupboard, putting it beside the one already on the counter. "I tell people to walk by the gate here, and then tell me fixed dogs don't bark or look fierce. Every one of the animals here, except for the very young or very sick, are spayed or neutered, and I'm sure you heard the racket when you drove up."

"I did," he agreed, with an answering laugh.

"Then I ask people what happens when their bitch or a neighbor's bitch goes into heat. We talk about the fights the dogs get into because of it, and how many animals die because of the wounds. I point out that while the dog is roaming the streets or the bitch is running, trying to escape the pack, they're not doing the work of guarding the house, so what's the use?"

"Does the logic work?"

She shrugged. "Sometimes. We take the wins where we can." The coffee was ready, and she turned off the machine. "Our best bet, I think, is with the kids."

Delano couldn't help noticing Mellie's straight-backed posture, the sweet flare of her hips beneath her long T-shirt, and had to drag his attention back to what she was saying as she poured their coffee.

"We take animals into the schools, especially at the primary level, to talk to the children about how to look after their animals. With the older ones, we talk about how they can tell if an animal is sick or in need of help." She crossed the kitchen in a couple steps and Delano took the proffered mug from her hand. It gave him a little thrill to note that although he thought she'd been ignoring him all this time, she obviously knew he took his coffee black, since she didn't offer cream or sugar. She went on: "The theory is that if we educate the children early on, we can change families' and communities' attitudes toward animals over time."

"And, in the meantime, you take in any of the animals that need help."

She'd already sat down across from him and she gave another shrug, accompanied this time with a little upward twist of her lips.

"As many as I can. Although I'm running out of space just now." Then, as though tired of the topic,

Mellie raised her eyebrows and asked, "So, what did you want to talk about?"

A little surprised by the swift change of subject, Delano took a sip of his coffee before saying, "I wanted to reiterate to you that there's no chance I'll be staying here in St. Eustace and taking over Dad's practice. My plan is, and always has been, to go back to Trinidad as soon as Dad's feeling better."

Mellie didn't answer right away. Instead, her gaze dropped to her hands, and Delano's followed. In the momentary silence, his words seemed to echo as he watched her turn the mug back and forth, back and forth between her fingers. It was as though she was searching for an appropriate response, and Delano's heart started pounding as he waited to hear what she'd say.

Was she thinking of their embrace the night before, rather than the clinic? He was honest enough to admit he'd be happy to know that. The attraction he felt toward her, that he was sure she felt toward him too, made him wish she'd say how disappointed she'd been when he left.

"That's..." She hesitated, eyes still downcast. "That's a shame."

Surprised by her response, Delano leaned back in his chair and the wave of emotion—hope and excitement—that welled inside him, rendered him mute.

CHAPTER NINE

AN EMOTION FLASHED across Delano's face that Mellie couldn't recognize and didn't know how to interpret. All she knew was that it sent a wave of goose bumps down her back, and made her heart turn over.

She'd been unsure about how to express what she thought, and now she realized how it might sound. That he might think she was speaking personally, rather than professionally, and a wave of embarrassment rose from her chest into her face.

Quickly, before he could comment or question her, she said, "Of course I'm hoping to carry on the practice when your father retires. I've put my all into it, helping to modernize and expand it, but that's just business. Your father means a lot to me—even more than the practice—and I know how happy it would make him if you decided to move back here and take over his work."

Delano nodded, leaning back in his chair, and his hooded regard made her want to squirm.

She'd spent far too long the night before reliving their kiss, to the point where she'd almost forgotten their frank and confiding conversation. If she were being totally honest, she'd have to admit that was where the real intimacy had bloomed between them.

She was ashamed to admit how judgmental she'd been when, realistically, she'd known very little about him. It brought to mind the way her mother acted, and Mellie had always promised herself never to emulate that behavior. Getting to know Delano had changed her attitude toward him, although part of her still wondered if she could trust him.

Her judgment of character was suspect, after all.

It was the kind of conundrum she really didn't need. But she was in the middle of it, whether she liked it or not, and had to find some way to navigate through to the best solution for them all.

How to manage that was the question.

Maybe the conversation would be easier if they weren't sitting so close together, and she had something to do with her hands other than hold her cup. Setting down her coffee, she stood up.

"Do you mind if I check on the kittens while we talk?" she asked, heading back into the living room without waiting for his agreement. "I've already fed them but might need to clean them up a bit before I leave for work."

He didn't reply, but she heard the scrape of the chair legs as he got up, and his measured footsteps as he followed her down the short hallway to the powder room door.

"It's a good thing I don't have a lot of visitors," she said, knowing she was babbling but not able to stop herself. "My guest bathroom seems to constantly be in use as a nursery."

Delano snorted: a sound she'd come to recognize denoted amusement, and somehow it made her relax, just a little.

When she pulled open the door, a tiny ball of black fur rocketed out, scooting between her feet then past Delano to disappear down the passageway.

"Gilligan!" They both shouted at the same time, just as an almighty crash sounded in the living room.

Mellie closed the bathroom door before rushing after Delano into the next room, and what she saw there brought her to a screeching halt.

The curtain rod across her large living room window was hanging down on one side, clearly brought down by the kitten, who was hanging onto the fabric with what looked to be one claw. The falling curtain had also knocked a metal lamp off a side table too.

"Good grief," Delano muttered, stepping over the lamp and reaching up for the kitten, who tried to scramble farther up the curtain but couldn't get his claw free. "Gilligan, you're more of a menace than your namesake was in the show."

For an instant, Mellie couldn't move, or even breathe. Delano was at full extension, both arms raised as he extricated the kitten from the curtain, and the view was mouthwatering. Shoulder and arm muscles flexed and his shirt rode up, revealing not just that perfect ass, but also a toothsome strip of dark, smooth skin above his low-slung jeans.

What was it about this man that caused her to burn inside, even while she knew it was best to stay away?

Closing her eyes for a moment and taking a deep breath, she sought calm although inside emotions tangled around her brain, making her wonder how to move forward. Delano drew her in by his magnetism and his seeming understanding of what drove her to rescue. Part of her wanted to run away before things went horribly wrong, but the other, larger part, wanted to get to know him intimately.

The dichotomy was enough to drive her a little insane.

A touch on her arm brought her back to herself, and her eyes flew open.

"You okay?"

He was close—too close—looking at her with such concern and curiosity, she felt herself blush furiously.

"Yes. Yes, I'm fine," she said. While she was trying to sound firm, she knew her voice was more breathless than she'd like. Sinking down onto the couch put some necessary distance between them. She'd been tempted to lean forward and kiss him.

Which was the last thing she should do.

"Listen," he said. Still holding the kitten close to his chest, he sat in the chair across from her. "I know you're thinking of my father's feelings, and I'll really think about what you said last night, but

St. Eustace isn't the place for me. When I left, I decided I wouldn't come back to live here, and that hasn't changed."

Looking down at her hands, Mellie chewed on her bottom lip, wanting to ask why, but knowing it wasn't any of her business.

"On a totally different subject," he said suddenly, making her look up in surprise. "Will there be a repeat of that kiss?"

All the breath left her lungs, and once more heat stained her cheeks and gathered low in her belly.

Damn him for making her feel like a giddy and unsophisticated schoolgirl!

"I don't know," she said, watching his expression—the slow upturn of those sinful lips, the gleam deep in his dark eyes—her heart rate spiking. "It probably wouldn't be wise."

His smile deepened into a grin, and he shook his head. "Wisdom is overrated, and a very minor part of my portfolio."

"I've learned to look at least twice before I leap," she rebutted. "We're working together. That complicates things."

"Not much," he replied. "Since I'll only be here for another week or so. Give me another excuse."

There were a hundred other reasons why kissing Delano should be on her no-no list, but for the life of her, when he looked at her with that smoldering intensity, she couldn't think of another one.

"It's not an excuse. I don't need an excuse not to kiss you." She made her voice as firm as she could, but it still wavered a little. "I need a reason to kiss you again."

He chuckled, and got to his feet in one lithe move. Holding Gilligan out to her, he said, "Well, I can give you a really good one, if you're interested."

Automatically taking the kitten and cuddling him close, Mellie met his gaze, and felt like she was drowning in it.

"What?" was all she could manage to ask, with her heart in her throat.

Delano bent, so his mouth was right beside her ear, and whispered, "It was superb."

Then, before she could catch enough breath to respond, he'd touched his lips to her cheek, and was on his way out the door.

"Dammit," she said to Gilligan, once Delano was gone. The kitten was looking at her with his bottle-green eyes, as if waiting for her verdict. "He's right."

Darn him!

Delano strode out, threading his way through the dogs, happily making a fuss over them the way they demanded. Going out through the gate, he unlocked the car then got in, grinning as he starting it, although his hands felt a little shaky.

Okay, so he'd done a complete one-eighty to what he'd intended when coming to Mellie's home, but that wasn't a bad thing. He had, after all, reiterated his determination not to stay and take over the practice, so Mellie could feel assured of her place there. As far as he knew, she had no reason not to believe him when he said he'd be going back to Trinidad.

But, even more importantly—to his mind anyway—he'd let her know he'd be more than happy to repeat their mind-blowing kiss. And take it further, if she was game.

Just the thought had his body hardening, and sent a wave of goose bumps along his back. He'd need a cold shower if he didn't stop thinking about Mellie. Those soft, full lips and silky skin. The way she'd pressed closer to him the night before and tangled her tongue with his in the most erotic of duels.

Whew.

She was one in a million, and if he was offered the privilege of an intimate, erotic encounter with her, there was no way he'd refuse.

His phone rang just as he drew up to his father's house and, recognizing his cousin's name and glad of the distraction, Delano answered it once he'd parked.

"Hey, Jason. What's up? Are you back?"

His cousin, who was an attaché to the minister of local government and culture, had been in Jamaica for a conference.

"Yes. Got in last night. Looking forward to seeing you. What you doing Saturday night? There's a big fundraiser out at Cable Farm. I thought we could go together. It'll be like old times."

"I hope not," Delano replied with a chuckle. "We drank way too much back in the day."

Jason laughed, the hearty sound buoying Delano's spirits even more, albeit in a very different way than his time with Mellie had. "We tore up the place, for sure. I'll make sure you don't overdo it at the fete. You're not as young as you used to be."

"Man, you're only a few months younger than me, so I don't get what you're yammering about."

"But I *am* younger than you, so there's that," his irrepressible cousin teased, making Delano laugh again. "I'll pick you up at about eight, if that works for you?"

"Sounds like a plan." It would be good to do something fun. "I'll see you then."

He was about to hang up and get out of the car when Jason said, "Wait, there's something else I need to speak to you about."

Sinking back into the driver's seat, Delano said, "Oh?"

"Yeah."

Jason paused, and the hair on the back of Delano's neck stirred. His cousin was usually both frank and completely self-assured. For him to hesitate didn't bode well for the conversation.

"Go on," Delano urged, wanting to get whatever was coming over with.

Jason's indrawn breath was loud enough for Delano to hear through the phone.

"For the last few years Uncle Milo has been talking about setting up a scholarship fund in Aunt Iris's memory, to help kids who want to go on to tertiary education. It was something he wanted to do long ago, but…"

When his cousin's voice faltered, Delano repeated, "But…?"

"Honestly, he wasn't in the financial position to do it." Jason's voice was firm, as if he'd come to a decision to tell it like it was. "After you left, the practice started to deteriorate a little at a time. Uncle Milo's heart wasn't in it. It's only since Mellie came to work with him, and started making improvements, that it's picked up again."

Delano leaned his head back against the seat, heartsore and swamped with guilt.

As if he didn't have enough of that on his plate.

"Anyway, he and I have been talking about how he wants the trust structured and other issues about the administration of it, and we're planning a big fundraiser next year." There was another pause, but brief this time. "Uncle Milo wants you to head it up."

"The fundraiser? Me?" He didn't know why he was so surprised, but shock had ricocheted through his body at his cousin's words.

"Not just the fundraiser. The entire thing."

CHAPTER TEN

MELLIE WAS CHECKING Rufus's incision site when Delano strode into the hospital, his expression stern and somehow abstracted. He acknowledged her presence with a grunt, and started pulling open drawers, one after the other, then closing them without taking anything out.

Not exactly the way she'd expected their next encounter would be, after his final sexy salvo that morning.

"What're you looking for?" she asked, finally.

"Hmm?" He didn't look up, but kept rifling through the suture drawer. "Exam room two needs some…" Stopping suddenly, he straightened and shook his head. "Dammit. I can't remember."

"Dude. You're not that old," she said, unable to suppress a chuckle, even though his behavior had her a bit worried. "What's going on?"

Delano closed the drawer and turned to face her with an interrogative look.

"Do you know that Dad's planning some type of memorial scholarship in Mum's name?"

Mellie nodded warily. "He's mentioned something recently—asking for fundraising ideas and stuff like that. Because your mother was a teacher, he thought it would be a fitting tribute to help kids who might not be able to afford a higher education."

He frowned. "Why am I only just hearing about it? And the fact that the practice was going downhill over the years?"

Rufus shifted on the examination table, and Mellie put both hands on him to keep him calm. She wished she could do the same to the confused and upset Delano.

"I don't know." That was the truth, if not what she thought. "Maybe your father didn't want to worry you while things were unsettled?"

Still with that fierce expression on his face, Delano shook his head.

"We both know that isn't it. He didn't tell me because he thought I didn't care."

What could she say to that?

"Well, he's told you now."

"That's the worst part," he growled. "He didn't tell me. My cousin Jason did instead."

"Oh." Delano still looked angry, but Mellie wasn't fooled. He was hurt.

Before she could think of something worthwhile to say, Delano slumped onto the stool across the table from her, and absently reached out to pet Rufus. As though the contact with the dog's fur and the little lick Rufus turned his head to bestow upon Delano's hand released some of his anger, Delano sighed.

"I'm at a loss, Mellie. Neither Dad nor Aunt

Eddie told me he was struggling to keep the clinic going. If I'd known..."

The unsaid words hung between them, and Mellie pursed her lips. It seemed unfair to press him, but until he faced his dilemma head-on, there was no way he could solve it.

"What?" she asked softly. "What would you have done? And be honest about it."

The silence between them was broken only by the whir of the ceiling fan and the sound of Rufus's breathing. Delano was looking down, his face creased into a frown. Then he looked up, and Mellie's heart ached at the torment in his eyes.

"I don't know."

Moved and sad for him, she put her hand over his and gave it a squeeze.

"And you won't ever know, because that moment is gone. If your father had told you, if you'd had to make a choice about what to do. If...if...if. The ifs will drive you crazy if you dwell on them too long. The truth is, this is a different moment in time, and the only way you're going to get any peace out of this trip is to sit down and talk honestly with your dad."

His mouth twisted slightly. "I'm out of practice doing that."

Mellie shrugged one shoulder. "Well, he's not the type of person who's going to bite your head off, or refuse to have a conversation. Not like my mom."

He turned his hand so he could hold hers, making her silly heart do a little flip.

"You're not in contact with your mother?"

"I reach out every now and then, but not really."

Now his expression was one of sympathy, and she was glad to give him something else to think about, and lift a little of the cloud hanging over his head.

"I'm sorry."

"Don't be. I had to come to the understanding that my mom chose not to be in my life, because her criteria for us having a relationship is too high for me to meet."

Curiosity seemed to war with his natural good manners, and the sight of him battling with the urge to ask questions made her smile.

"You can ask me whatever you want," she said. "Just not right now. The clinic's about to open, and Rufus doesn't know it yet, but he's going home today. Mr. Brixton is coming for him this morning."

She lifted Rufus down from the table, placing him gently on the floor. With one hand under his abdomen, she kept the dog standing.

"That's good," Delano said after a little pause, as though he was still thinking through their conversation. "Hopefully that'll improve his mood."

"Both their moods, I think." Keeping her voice cheerful was a bit of a chore since she suddenly felt as though she'd run an emotional marathon. "Mr. Brixton looked so sad when he had to leave him after the operation."

At Mellie's urging Rufus took a few tentative

steps, looking up at her with the saddest puppy dog eyes imaginable.

"You got this, Rufus," she said, letting go of his belly so he was moving on his own, albeit jerkily. "You can do it."

And, as she led the dog out of the exam room, Mellie touched Delano's shoulder, saying, "You got this too. Remember, the future doesn't have to be the same as the past. Have that chat with your father..."

"If he'll let me.

"He'll let you," she replied. "He's missed having you in his life, whether you want to acknowledge that or not."

Then she took Rufus out to do his business, so when Mr. Brixton came to pick him up he'd be ready to go.

Delano found himself considering Mellie's words all morning, in between seeing patients. The volume of clients was still high enough to keep them both busy, but when he heard Mr. Brixton was there to pick up Rufus, he made sure to take a few minutes to say goodbye to the dog.

"He looks so much better," Mr. Brixton said, smiling widely as his hand first stroked his dog's head, then scratched behind one floppy ear. "And he's walking on his own."

Rufus's tail was wagging for the first time since he'd come in, his eyes were noticeably brighter, and where before his nose had been dull and dry, now it shone.

"It'll take him a while to fully regain his balance and agility," Mellie told the older gentleman. "But dogs generally do well after an amputation, and the best place for him now is at home with you. Being back in familiar surroundings with his favorite person will be better than any medicine we can give him."

She had such an easy way about her, and a really lovely voice. Remembering the husky timbre of it after they'd kissed gave him all kinds of naughty ideas he hoped to be able to put into practice.

Even in the midst of his personal turmoil, there was no ignoring the effect Mellie had on him, but it was up to her whether their relationship ever got to the next level. Not only wasn't he the type to push, but he also respected her cautious attitude. If she decided it wasn't worth the potential problems, he'd have to respect that.

Not that he'd like it.

Quickly saying farewell to both Rufus and his owner, Delano excused himself to see his next patient. But he kept listening to Mellie as she gave Mr. Brixton instructions about how to care for his dog until he couldn't hear her anymore.

Bearing in mind what Mellie had said earlier that day, about how he might be able to move forward with his father, Delano took a moment between patients to call home.

When he asked Aunt Eddie if he could come back there for lunch, she replied, "Of course, boy. Plenty of food here."

He got to the house as his father was sitting down at the kitchen table.

"Just in time," Dad said, giving Delano a sideways glance. "I was afraid you'd be late and Eddie would make me wait until you got here."

"Thank goodness Delano keeps better time than you do," was Eddie's tart response. "The number of nights dinner got cold waiting on you…"

"All right. All right." Dad tried to sound put upon, but he was smiling, since they all knew it was true.

Delano washed his hands and helped Aunt Eddie carry the dishes of chicken, boiled green bananas, cassava, yam and salad to the table. Impossible not to feel a pang of nostalgia as he surveyed the food. His father, unlike many of his countrymen, didn't eat a lot of rice with his meals, preferring ground provisions, like the cassava, and other kinds of carbohydrates. It was how Delano had grown up, and he realized now that he'd missed it.

There was so much to love about his homeland. And so much pain associated with it too.

After his father had blessed the meal, and Aunt Eddie passed around the dishes, his father said, "I haven't had a chance to ask you how obedience class went."

That was a safe enough subject, so Delano gave

them a rundown of what had happened, making his father laugh.

"Did you really fall down?" he asked, still chuckling.

"Flat-flat," Delano assured him. "On my back, looking up at the sky, wondering how I'd gotten myself into such a position."

"I don't know what you're laughing about, Milo," Aunt Eddie said, her lips twitching as she tried to hold back her own amusement. "Remember the time the bull chased you into the pond?"

That set the tone for the meal, and although Delano hadn't asked his father about either the trust or what had happened with the clinic, it felt like a success. They hadn't really spoken much since Delano arrived, and now it was as if they'd partway crossed the barrier between them.

On impulse, Delano asked, "How about coming to obedience class next Wednesday, even just for a little while? We can set you up in the pavilion, where you can see everything, and get you a taxi home if you don't want to stay until the end."

He wasn't sure where the suggestion sprang from, but the pleasure on his father's face let him know it was the right one.

"I will," Dad said, smiling broadly.

"Give him a megaphone," the irrepressible Aunt Eddie muttered. "So he can boss you around from the sidelines."

"Cho," was his father's response, but he was still smiling.

After lunch was over, Aunt Eddie got a telephone call and went out onto the veranda to take it, leaving Delano and his father alone at the table.

That was as good a time as any, Delano thought.

"Dad, I spoke to Jason today."

"Oh, yes? I didn't know he was back already."

There was no change in his father's demeanor.

"Just got back today. He was telling me about the memorial trust you want to set up."

Dad definitely stiffened, and his gaze searched Delano's face.

Then he huffed.

"I told your cousin I'd talk to you myself when I was ready," he said, the corners of his lips turning down.

"But I don't know why you wouldn't have spoken to me about it from the start—when you first had the idea."

With a little shrug, his father leaned back in his chair, trying to look nonchalant, even though his gaze stayed fixed on Delano's face.

"It was just an idea. And Jason would know who I needed to talk to if I decided to set it up. Lawyers and so forth."

A spurt of annoyance made Delano lean back in his own chair, trying to match his father's casualness. If Dad didn't want to talk about it—be honest with him—then what was the use of even trying?

Then, like a whisper in his ear, he heard Mellie's voice: *The future doesn't have to be the same as the past...*

And neither did the present. But one of them would have to break the habit of silence and deflection if there was to be any chance of making a change.

Clearly, it would have to be him.

"Dad, I couldn't help you navigate the laws here, but I would be able to give you some idea of what it entails to set up the kind of foundation you're thinking of, although mine's on a pretty small scale."

His father's gaze sharpened.

"Oh?"

Putting his elbows on the table, getting physically closer to his dad, Delano nodded.

"I set up one, myself, a few years ago. Once a year it pays for sports equipment for a primary school—cricket bats and pads, or soccer balls and cleats, that sort of thing—up to the limit of what the fund can afford. The schools apply, showing their need, and I have to pick one to benefit. That's the hardest part, to be honest."

Eyes wide now, Dad stared, and Delano would have laughed at the way his mouth moved and nothing came out, if the moment itself wasn't so important.

"You have a…?"

Delano nodded. "A foundation? Yes. Took a while to get going. Stella wasn't on board with it, so saving and investing a reasonable amount of funds was the work of years."

His ex-wife had hated the fact that he was saving money for a cause she didn't think was terribly important. Or, in hindsight, maybe what had upset her was not being in on the planning stage. Looking back, he realized he'd downplayed the importance of it to her.

He'd held his pain close, denying her access to those emotions that had shaped him into the man he was.

It was the only way he knew how to deal with them.

But that was in the past, and now he needed to move forward into the future and rebuild a relationship with his father. Even if it meant opening up the wounds they shared.

Swallowing hard against the lump forming in his throat, he said, "I called it the E.G. Foundation."

His father blinked, and his mouth moved again, this time not with shock but in an effort to speak.

"Everard Gopaul." Dad's voice wavered, and he lifted a hand to cover his eyes for a second. When it fell away, Delano could see the moisture in his father's eyes, and his own prickled too. "Everard loved sports. I remember him racing down the soccer pitch, leaving everyone in his dust." His father reached across the table and squeezed Delano's forearm tight. "That's a perfect memorial, son."

And for the first time in too many years to count, Delano felt connected to his father again.

CHAPTER ELEVEN

FRIDAY WAS THE kind of day that made Mellie want to go back to bed from the moment she woke up. Johnny Luck had an asthma attack first thing in the morning, one bad enough that it had Mellie rushing him to the hospital. After promising him she'd be back to check on him as soon as possible, she returned to the shelter to take care of the animals on her own.

Knowing it was going to make her late to the office, she called Delano once she thought he'd be awake to let him know what was happening.

"No problem," was all he said.

After hanging up, she started on her feeding chores, but before she'd gotten more than halfway through, she'd been surprised by a knock on the gate.

It was Delano, dressed in a pair of old jeans and a T-shirt that fit him way too snugly for her equilibrium.

"What are you doing here?" she asked, after she'd waved him in.

"I figured you'd need some help," he replied, a broad grin on his face. "Many hands make light work, as Aunt Eddie is fond of saying."

"Well," she said, reluctantly, "I'm not going to turn you away. I appreciate the help."

But in a way he made her work harder, because she found herself watching him as much as concentrating on what she needed to do.

Although he hadn't reiterated his invitation to indulge in more kisses, the thought of it—and what else might happen between them—hadn't left her mind, at all. At the most inconvenient moments she found herself remembering, and was awash with pleasure and need.

Yet, they got everything done in time for both of them to make it to the clinic before it opened, even though Mellie stopped at the hospital to see Johnny.

"I didn't get a chance to ask you earlier," Delano said when they met up in the office later that morning. "What plans do you have for the weekend?"

The question made heat rush through her veins.

Was he inviting her out?

Mellie resolutely pushed that thought aside.

"I have a meeting of the shelter board this evening, to finalize the plans for the spay and neuter clinic next week. Then, if Johnny isn't feeling better, I'll have my work cut out for me on Saturday and Sunday, as well as laundry and all the other stuff I need to do." She couldn't help sighing. "Not exactly how I'd planned to spend this weekend, but that's how it goes sometimes."

"If you need my help, just call." He was still smiling, although he was already shaking his head.

"Don't be so darned independent that you wear yourself out unnecessarily."

Wishing he wasn't being so nice to her—since it just made her want to melt—Mellie nodded. "I'll call, if I need help."

Which totally meant she had no intention of calling. It wouldn't be the first time she'd managed the shelter feeding and cleaning on her own, and it was doubtful it would be the last.

"What do you have planned?" she asked in return, curious, although she knew she shouldn't be.

"Spending tonight with Dad, whether he likes it or not." That made Mellie chuckle, but she was glad he was making the effort. "Then going out with a cousin of mine tomorrow night. We haven't hung out together in a long time. Not since the last time he came to Trinidad, about four years ago."

"Nice," was all she had time to say before they were deluged with patients, including a couple of emergencies, that had them both staying later than either one had planned.

She'd arranged with one of the clinic workers to go by her house to take care of the animals since Johnny, although he was out of the hospital, needed to rest. Mellie only had enough time to get to the restaurant where the shelter board was meeting, and then only because she didn't go home to change.

The directors were all there ahead of her, sipping drinks and chatting. Amity got up to hug her, but it was Janice Gopaul that Mellie looked at first. The older woman appeared tired, her face thinner and a bit drawn. And during the meeting, when it was mentioned that Delano was on the roster for the clinic, Janice's gaze dropped to the glass she was holding and her lips tightened.

It took them a couple of hours to get everything hashed out and, as they all got up to leave, Mellie thought Janice might hang back to talk, but the other woman said a terse good-night and left immediately.

It was Amity who walked out with Mellie, slinging her arm around Mellie's shoulders. "Hey, listen. I have an extra ticket to the party up at Cable Farm tomorrow night. Come with me, nuh?"

"I wish I could." Mellie stifled a yawn behind her hand, exhausted at the thought of going home to look after her house dogs. "But Johnny had an asthma attack this morning, and I'll probably have to take care of all the animals by myself tomorrow. I'll be too tired to go out afterward."

"That never stopped you before," her friend teased, bumping her hip. "You getting old?"

"Yeah, maybe."

"Stop it! You have to come. It's for a good cause, and you haven't been out in ages."

Knowing her friend wouldn't stop until she at least agreed to consider it, Mellie gave in.

"I'll try, but I won't know until the afternoon whether I'll be able to or not."

But Amity crowed as if she'd already got her way, and did a little calypso shimmy on the way to her car.

By the time Mellie finally fell into bed that night, she had already decided not to go to the party. If Delano was going out with his cousin, it stood to reason they might end up at Cable Farm. It was one of the biggest parties of the year. With the attraction she could no longer ignore simmering between them, seeing Delano there, socially, might lead her to do something silly.

Like invite him home with her.

And if he wasn't there, she'd be disappointed.

Somehow, at that moment, it was a toss-up as to which seemed worse.

The following morning, the dogs barking and people talking were what woke her. Squinting at her phone, she realized she'd overslept, and she rushed to pull on some clothes and peek outside.

Delano and Johnny were in the dog pen, laughing together like old friends.

Letting the house dogs out, she decided to make some coffee before going out there and giving both of them hell, but by the time she'd taken the first sip of caffeine, she'd lost the urge to quarrel.

"What are you both doing?" she called when she was within earshot, causing the men to turn to face her.

"Just cleaning up, as always, Dr. Mellie." Johnny grinned, exposing an expanse of gum.

"Aren't you supposed to be resting?"

That earned her a rude sound from Johnny.

"I fine now, Dr. Mellie. No fuss mi."

Turning her gaze to Delano she gave him a narrow-eyed glare.

"And don't you have other things to do?"

He grinned, one of those winning smiles he utilized so well.

"Not really. I've already taken Baldur for his run, and had breakfast with Dad. Nothing else on the agenda right now, at all."

Mellie sighed.

"And I suppose you're going to want coffee on top of everything, huh?"

She said it as if grudgingly but smiled at the same time, letting him know she was both grateful for his help and forgiving of his assumption that she needed it.

Delano tried to look rueful, but failed. His eyes were twinkling and crinkled at the corners, and he couldn't control the upward tilt of his lips.

"I don't want to put you out…"

She snorted, and headed back toward the cottage, saying over her shoulder, "The temerity! Just for that, meet me in the kennels. I'm putting you on cleanup duty."

And his shout of laughter made her grin, knowing he wouldn't see the evidence of her amusement.

Taking care of the animals in the shelter was hard work, but Delano didn't mind, particularly as it had become easier and easier to open up to her about his journey with his father. While he couldn't yet bring himself to speak about their conversation about

Everard, just telling her that the ice had been broken was a big step for him.

"What did you end up doing last night?" she asked, after saying she'd fallen into bed and was asleep as soon as her head hit the pillow.

"Your father came by with Mr. Andy, and we ended up playing dominoes."

She sent him an amused glance. "Not the type of pastime I would recommend for a man who's supposed to be resting. Not the way your father plays, anyway. He always gets so worked up."

Delano chuckled with her. "Aunt Eddie read us the riot act before we started. Said if she heard tiles banging on the table or raised voices, she'd put a stop to the game. And Dad was happy because he and your father won six-two. No need for him to get upset, although I'm sure he'd have been even happier if it was six-love."

"Of course he would," she agreed. "And Daddy would have been too, but at least your ego was spared that humiliation."

"I'm not as radical as they are when it comes to winning," he replied, honestly. "Mr. Andy wasn't happy with me, but obviously keeping on Aunt Eddie's good side was more important than expressing his frustrations."

"Oh, hell yes," Mellie agreed with a snort. "Everyone knows your aunt isn't to be trifled with. My father loves her, but freely admits to being completely intimidated by her. He says although she's younger, she used to keep him and Dr. Milo in line even when they were children."

"I can believe that."

"It must be nice to have friends of such long standing," she said, a wistful note in her voice. "As close as family, but even more treasured because you chose them, you know?"

Delano thought of Everard, and sadness swamped him; it wasn't as sharp as it used to be, but still there. Then he pushed it away, wanting simply to enjoy the day with Mellie, rather than being bogged down with regrets.

"You don't have anyone like that?" he asked, hoping she wouldn't turn the question back on him.

"No." The way she spoke suggested it was all she was going to say on the subject. A complete sentence. So it was a bit of a surprise when she continued, "When I was very young, we moved around too much. And even when we settled in Chicago— after Mom married Tony—I didn't really know how to make friends." She paused, a thoughtful expression pulling her eyebrows together. "To be honest, my mother was too unpredictable for me to feel comfortable bringing people to the house. It was too much of a risk.

"And now, ever since I got in touch with Daddy, she's been unhappy with me. Her criteria for us having a relationship is that I go back to the States and not keep in contact with my father."

"That's harsh," Delano said, shocked and saddened.

Mellie just shrugged, though. "If you met her, you'd understand. She wants everything her way. Thank goodness I realized a long time ago that I deserved to make my own decisions, whether she approves or not, or whether they turned out to be good or bad."

Trying to lighten the mood, he said, "I can't see you making any really bad choices. You seem really methodical and levelheaded, like you have everything together."

That made her burst out laughing. "You have no idea just how terrible some of my decisions have been." Before he could ask, she held up a hand, and continued, "Maybe one day I'll tell you about it, but not today." She looked out into the sunshine and said, "It's too nice a day to go down that road."

"Okay," he teased, "I'll wait until a rainy day, then ask you."

"And if it's gloomy enough, I just might tell you. Where are you and your cousin going tonight?"

He followed her lead, turning down this new conversational path with her.

"Some charity do, out on a farm."

"Up at Cable Farm," she said, nodding. "My best friend, Amity, invited me too, but I haven't decided whether to go or not yet."

"Well, if you decide to come, save me a dance."

He made an effort to sound casual, but when she slanted him an enigmatic glance his body heated. For a long moment their gazes clashed, and the electricity sparking hot and arousing between them singed him down to the bone.

Then she turned away, and he thought he heard her take a deep inhale.

"We'll see," was all she said.

And he had to content himself with that.

CHAPTER TWELVE

MELLIE DILLYDALLIED ALL day about whether to go to the Cable Farm party. While she'd pretty much decided from the night before not to go, there was no escaping the fact that knowing Delano would be there made it more appealing.

Especially if he made good on his request for a dance.

Just the thought made her break out in goose bumps.

Of course, maybe he was thinking of a fast calypso or reggae tune, but her brain kept insisting on imagining a slow, smoochy number, where they'd be locked in each other's arms.

There was no mistaking the rising awareness flowing back and forth between them, which had reached new heights that day as they worked side by side. More than once their gazes had locked, and Mellie hadn't been able to ignore the heat gathering beneath her skin and in her core.

It was probably just because she was in the midst of a sexual drought, she told herself. The last relationship she'd had was two years ago, and calling it a *relationship* was really stretching it. The truth was, she didn't have time to devote to being a part of a functioning couple, between work, the shelter and all the other projects she had going on. She'd gone out with Rafe over the space of three months, slept with him a few times, but when he'd started complaining about her lack of availability, she'd had to call it quits.

And, in reality, she had felt only a brief moment of guilt and sadness.

She'd enjoyed the companionship, but hadn't been that into him, no matter how handsome and nice he'd been.

There certainly hadn't been the sparks she felt whenever she was around Delano.

Telling herself it was ridiculous to even consider getting involved with Dr. Milo's son hadn't worked. In fact, the more she argued with herself about it, the less ludicrous it sounded.

She had no time or wish to be in a serious relationship, and Delano had assured her he was only here for a short time. If he was interested in a brief, sex-only relationship, it would suit her fine.

Without the worry of getting too emotionally involved, she could simply enjoy him and not fret about his trustworthiness.

Not that she mistrusted him the way she had at first. The more she got to know him, the less she believed her initial impressions and assumptions were correct. His belief that his father didn't want him around hinted at a deeper issue Mellie wasn't privy to, but was desperately curious about.

But she was the last person to delve into other people's pains and sorrows, knowing she didn't really want to share her own. Only her father knew fully what had happened back in Miami, since he'd been the one to help her clean up the mess she'd found herself in. Dr. Milo knew a part of the story, but he was like a clam when it came to gossip, which Mellie completely appreciated.

There was no way she'd have been able to build her new life here in St. Eustace if everyone had known the shambles she'd made of her previous one. It would have been too embarrassing.

Amity was overjoyed when Mellie called to let her know she'd go with her to the party.

"You want me to pick you up?" Mellie asked her friend, since she could drive past Amity's apartment on her way to the farm, while Amity would have to go way out of her way to get Mellie.

"Better we drive separately," Amity replied. "Since I know you're going to want to leave before I'm ready to go home. Meet me here, and we'll drive in convoy."

Laughing, Mellie agreed. Amity would probably be among the last to leave the party, while Mellie had to be up early in the morning.

When she arrived at Amity's place later that evening, her friend gave a *whoop* of appreciation.

"Look at you, Miss Thing. I haven't seen you dressed up like this in forever. I knew that outfit was perfect for you, remember?"

Mellie felt the heat rise into her face, but tried to act nonchalant.

"Yes, I remember. I just felt like looking pretty,"

she said, as though it hadn't taken her over an hour to figure out what to wear. What would turn Delano's head enough that he'd make a move, or give her the opening to make one herself?

Finally she'd chosen a bright coral pink dress, the fabric as ethereal as a sigh. From the shoestring strap that held it up and gathered the material along the neckline, it fell to midthigh, leaving her shoulders bare. On the hanger it looked frumpy, making Mellie wonder why she bought it each time she saw it in the closet, but when she put it on, and saw the way it caressed her curves, she remembered.

Amity's perfectly shaped eyebrows rose.

"You always look pretty, even in scrubs," she said stoutly. "But I can see you put in extra effort tonight. For anyone in particular?"

"Myself." Then, knowing her friend wouldn't stop until Mellie came clean about why her cheeks were now burning hot, she added, "To give me courage."

Amity snapped her fingers. "Delano Logan, right?"

"Why'd you jump to that conclusion?"

Amity held up her hand and counted off on her fingers each point as she made them.

"One—he's gorgeous. Two—he's available. Three—he's the only man you've been in close contact with recently."

"That you know of," Mellie interjected, earning herself an eyeroll from her friend.

"That I know of for certain. Four—he's just your type—smart, jovial, hardworking, oh, and did I mention gorgeous?"

"That's twice now," Mellie muttered.

"I rest my case," Amity replied, the smugness in her voice making Mellie chuckle.

"You missed a point, though," Mellie said as Amity locked her front door, and they went down the steps to the car park.

"Which point?"

"He'll only be here for another week or so."

Amity stopped and shook her head.

"One of these days you're going to have to get over your commitment-phobia, Mellie."

"But today is not that day," Mellie rebutted. "Today, all I'm interested in is seeing if I can get Delano Logan into my bed."

"And more power to you," came Amity's reply, although she was still shaking her head, as though in disbelief.

Cable Farm was a coffee plantation in the hills, the main house built of stone and registered as a historical building by the Ministry of Culture. It had been repaired and refurbished back to its former glory, and was operated as a bed-and-breakfast by the owner, who lived in a smaller house on the property. For the charity function the house was lit up. There were tables and chairs on the lawn and, from there, down a short flight of stairs on the terraced hillside, a wooden dance floor had been erected.

Mellie and Amity paused on the lawn, surveying the crowd of people already in attendance.

"My parents are here somewhere," Amity said,

glancing at the occupied tables. "But I'm guessing they'll leave right after they've eaten. Is your father coming?"

"He has a polo match tomorrow, so no. When I asked him, he said he was too old to be feting the night before a match."

"Sounds reasonable. You see your guy yet?"

It was on the tip of her tongue to say Delano wasn't her guy, but it was too late to close the barn door on that one.

"No."

"The bar," Amity said, with her usual determination. "And even if he isn't there, I want a drink."

As they strolled along, returning greetings and hugs with all the people they knew, suddenly there he was, and Mellie's breath hitched when she saw the way he was looking at her. As he strode toward her, he was smiling, but it looked more predatory than amused, and his eyes gleamed behind half-closed lids.

"Mmm-hmm," murmured Amity, just loud enough for the sound to reach Mellie's ear. "You're definitely getting lucky tonight."

And all Mellie could do was hope the evening shadows hid the rush of color to her cheeks.

Delano could hardly believe his eyes.

From the first moment he'd seen Mellie he'd been attracted to her, even though she was threatening him with a machete. In his eyes she was beautiful, and had only grown more so as he'd spent time with and gotten to know her.

But tonight…

Tonight she was radiant. Sexy. Sinfully sensual.

Her pink dress flowed around her body, touching it the way he longed to—softly caressing with each move. Through some feminine alchemy she appeared to be naked beneath the silky fabric, as each and every curve and dip was alternately revealed and concealed. The light evening breeze added to that illusion, making the dress froth and swing with each gust.

It took everything he had within not to grab and kiss her, before dragging her away from the party and all the prying eyes around them.

All he could think about was running his hands all over her, bringing her to full, shivering arousal, before stripping her naked and making love to her in every way possible.

The intensity of his reaction pulled him up short, though. It wasn't his way to come on strong. It never had been. So he resigned himself to waiting, and letting her set the pace, if that was what she wanted.

But that didn't mean that he couldn't express his appreciation.

He walked right up to her, hardly aware there was someone else standing beside her and completely forgetting his cousin Jason, who was keeping pace with him as he made a beeline to Mellie.

"You look fabulous," he told her, wanting to

touch her in some way, but hesitating because he wasn't sure he wouldn't do something ridiculous, like full-on kiss her. "Absolutely stunning."

Rather than slough him off as he expected, Mellie gave him a long look, her lips pursed in a winsome pout.

"Thank you," she murmured. "I felt like dressing up a bit this evening."

He couldn't even reply, because as she spoke she ran her hand along her side, molding that magical fabric to her curves, and making his palm itch with the urge to follow her example.

"Jason," came Amity's half amused, half resigned voice, "Come let's get a drink. I know when I'm not wanted."

"Me too," was the laughing answer, and Delano was hardly aware of them leaving until Mellie's gaze broke from his and followed the other couple as they walked away.

"Oh, I don't think I've ever met your cousin," she said. "And you didn't introduce us."

"I'll do it later." Hooking an arm around her waist, he turned her toward the dance floor. The DJ was playing calypso, and while it wasn't the ideal musical genre for how he was feeling, there was still an opportunity to pull Mellie close every now and then. "I'm claiming my dance now, before anyone else beats me to it."

"There's no rush." When she laid a hand on his chest, he was sure she could feel his heart thumping through his shirt. "Let's wait until they play something a little slower."

That was when Delano was absolutely sure that she wanted the same thing he did. And that some-time soon, perhaps even tonight, he'd get to know Mellie as intimately as he craved.

Shifting his hand so it lay against the small of her back, trying to ignore the heat of her body through the thin material, he cleared his throat and asked, "How about a drink, then, and an intro to my cousin?"

"Sure." She slanted him a glance from the cor-ner of her eye, her smile almost sly. This was a dif-ferent Mellie again from the one he'd experienced earlier. A little more subdued, definitely with an increased sultriness quotient. "There definitely is no need to hurry."

His heart stopped, the double entendre making his entire body tighten.

But her voice was serene when she continued, "Come on. I see Kiah Langdon and his wife, Mina. You'll like them. They're really fun."

And he was forced to marshal every ounce of control and nod, following meekly after her, when what he really wanted to do was throw her over his shoulder and race away.

Get her somewhere private so he could kiss that tempting smile right off her lips.

CHAPTER THIRTEEN

MELLIE KNEW SHE was teasing Delano, both with her flirtation and her determination to wait, despite wanting him almost unbearably already. The truth of the matter was she had two very good reasons to delay what she now considered to be the inevitable conclusion of the night.

Him. Her. Together. In bed.

If he'd asked, she'd have told him that although he was still a stranger to many of the people at the party, she wasn't. Also, by night's end, because of his father's popularity, anyone who wasn't acquainted with him certainly would know who Delano was if they wanted to.

It stood to reason that if they ran out of the party before it even properly got going, both his father and hers would hear about it by the following morning. If she and Delano decided to sleep together and prolong their affair for the rest of the time he was in St. Eustace, that would be soon enough to run the gauntlet of parental scrutiny. But since they hadn't even got to that point yet, Mellie didn't see any advantage in getting either Dr. Milo or her dad too excited about their offspring falling into bed together.

The second reason was that she realized the anticipation would only make the entire situation sweeter.

The little touches they exchanged. The heated glances. The knowledge that soon whatever erotic fantasies they were weaving in their heads stood a good chance of coming true. All those heightened the sensation of a monumental event on the horizon, slowly building, waiting for the right instance to burst forth into pleasure.

And she liked that. A lot.

So she took him over to where a group from the hospital was standing, integrating into the crowd and introducing him.

"You know Kiah, from obedient class," she said. "And this is his wife, Dr. Mina Haraldson. This mischief-maker is Dr. Gen Broussard—one of our best surgeons—and her husband, Zach Lewin, who all work at Port Michael Public Hospital. This is Dr. Milo's son, Delano."

Gen laughed, and swatted Mellie on the arm.

"How dare you introduce me that way?" she asked, her Southern accent enhanced by a newly acquired island swing. "Please don't listen to her, Dr. Logan. I'm an angel, as everyone else will attest to."

"Not if we don't want to be struck by lightning," her husband muttered, earning a glare. But when everyone else chuckled, Gen was laughing with them.

This was one of the reasons she'd chosen this particular group. Their levity and comfort with each other helped ease the tension between her and Delano somewhat. Amity and Jason also came over, and the hilarity increased exponentially. Gen and Amity were friends, and teased each other unmercifully, and there was no shortage of comical stories told.

"Did Gen have a stroke?" Delano whispered into Mellie's ear at one point, giving her goose bumps as his warm breath wafted across her cheek, and his delicious scent ignited her olfactory senses.

Leaning close so her lips were against his ear in turn, and resting her hand on his arm, she murmured, "Bell's palsy."

There was no mistaking the shiver that traveled through Delano's body, and Mellie couldn't help smiling to herself as she rejoined the general conversation.

They chatted, laughed and danced, and the entire group commandeered a table when dinner was served. Although surrounded by all the others, and sometimes separated from him, Mellie was constantly and completely aware of where Delano was at all times.

And whenever she ventured a glance in his direction, it was often to find his gaze squarely on her, as well.

The night took on an almost dreamlike aura. Mellie couldn't remember when she'd had so good a time, or felt so confident and beautiful. Despite them both seemingly making an effort to not appear to be together, she and Delano orbited each other, connected by a thread of attraction.

She'd nursed a glass of red wine all evening, but it struck her, suddenly, that she felt tipsy with happiness. And while she could freely acknowledge to herself that Delano had a lot—more than a lot—to do with that, there was also a part of her that insisted she remember not to get in too deep.

That while she no longer distrusted him the way she had in the beginning, there was no upside to risking more than her physical self with this man.

And she was determined to share nothing else but that.

It turned out that Kiah's grandmother, Miss Pearl, and Delano's aunt Eddie were old friends from church, and that led to more jokes and laughter, as the two men compared stories.

This was a Delano Mellie hadn't experienced before. Although he'd seemed charming and sociable from the beginning, she realized he hadn't been truly relaxed. Not like he was now, surrounded by uncomplicated company.

Just then, as Kiah was telling Zach about Miss Eddie, and the way she and his own grandmother seemed to know everything happening in Port Michael, Delano looked across at her, and Mellie's heart stopped.

Beneath the laughter in his gaze was heat to match her own, and the intensity of it made her breath catch deep in her chest.

Looking away was difficult, but imperative if

she didn't want everyone else at the table to know how much she desired him.

Amity nudged Mellie.

"Isn't that your dad's neighbor, Mr. Ramos?"

Thankful for the interruption, Mellie looked in the direction she was pointing, spotting the elderly man walking toward the car park.

"Oh, yes. I should go speak to him."

Without sparing Delano another glance, she got up from the table and took off after her father's friend, glad to have a chance to catch her breath, away from Delano.

Delano watched Mellie hurry after the older gentleman, enjoying the view of her swinging hips in that bewitching dress.

The woman he'd seen this evening was the one he'd been longing to interact with. Mellie had laughed and teased and shone, bright as the Caribbean sun at midday. Her beauty and personality had dazzled him all over again, but whereas before he'd been on the outside and looking in, tonight she'd drawn him right in.

And he couldn't get enough of it.

He'd felt at home with her in a way he had to acknowledge he hadn't experienced in a long time. Oh, it was easy to be cordial and make casual friendships that didn't take much to sustain. He'd been doing it all his life, and had no complaints. Yet, somehow, tonight he'd had to face the fact that he'd actually been missing out on something important.

Just like he'd missed out on being an integral part of his family too.

"She looks gorgeous tonight, doesn't she?"

Amity's question jerked him out of his ruminations, and he turned to find she'd slid into the seat beside him and was watching him with a sly smile on her face.

"She always looks gorgeous," he said, before he'd thought it through.

The grin Amity sent his way let him know she'd made note of his reply and happily filed it away.

"I'm sure she'd be glad to hear you say so." They both watched silently for a moment as Mellie looped her arm through that of Mr. Ramos and the two of them strolled toward the parking area. "I'm glad to see her enjoying herself so much. She's a wonderful woman, and friend, but she works so hard she doesn't have much fun."

"I'm surprised," Delano said, tearing his gaze away from Mellie and giving his full attention to her friend. "With a crowd like this, I'd have thought she'd be out all the time."

Amity shrugged lightly. "We try, but she gives her all to everything she does, and she's fiercely independent to boot. Often that means running herself almost into the ground to get everything done, because she's trying to do it all herself. Doesn't leave much time for parties or even socializing much."

"Hmm. And she's planning to take on even more—either with taking over from Dad at the clinic, or expanding the shelter."

"She'll manage," Amity said with conviction. "I don't want you to get the idea that she's not capable, because she is. We're putting plans in place—I'm on the board of the shelter—for the eventual expansion. It's set up as a not-for-profit, and runs on mostly donations, but Mellie has made some impressive connections and there's a chance for some sponsorships and other moneymakers in the works."

"How long can she go on where she is, before she has to expand?"

"She's already there," Amity replied. "The shelter is just about at capacity. The outreach programs can continue, of course, but unless she gets a bigger place, or gets a bunch of animals adopted, Mellie's going to have to halt intake."

He shouldn't care, but Amity's words struck him like a blow to the solar plexus. From seeing her with the animals, from the kittens the taxi man had brought to the clinic, and the dogs, other cats, goat kids, and the pigs Jane and Bingley, he knew rescue was where her heart lay.

"I don't see her stopping. If an animal needs help, she'll do what she can to take it in," he said. After all, he'd seen that with his own eyes in the case of the kittens, which she'd taken into her house since the cattery nursery was already full.

Amity's lips quirked. "You know her better than I gave you credit for."

For some unfathomable reason, her words made heat rush up from his chest and into his face. Thankfully, she glanced away just then, and he saw her frown.

"Oh, darn it."

When he followed her gaze, he saw Mellie standing on the edge of the car park, speaking to a man who definitely wasn't the elderly Mr. Ramos. He was about the same height as Mellie, and was standing way too close, his face just inches from hers.

The sight caused such a rush of annoyance that he had to swallow to speak lightly.

"Someone doesn't appreciate the concept of personal space, does he?"

Amity snorted. "And Mellie doesn't much care for him. Look at how she's leaning away. I wonder if he has bad breath too?"

It was Delano's turn to snort, but there was no amusement in the sound. His annoyance was edging toward anger.

"Who is he, anyway?"

"Martin McGovern. An American working in the accounts department of one of the new hotels. Mellie went on one date with him about four months ago but didn't like him. He's been trying to get her to go out with him again ever since." Amity nudged him with her elbow, hard enough that Delano grunted. "You should go rescue her."

"I'm pretty sure Mellie can rescue herself," he

replied, but he was already on his feet, and Amity laughed as he walked away.

Plastering a smile on his face, he strode up to Mellie and slung an arm around her waist. Startled, she turned to look up at him, and he planted a smacking kiss right on her lips. When he let his mouth linger on hers, she didn't pull away.

Instead, she leaned into his embrace, and Delano almost forgot what it was he was trying to achieve.

Only when he heard the other man clear his throat did Delano pull back.

Not releasing his hold on Mellie's waist, he looked at the accountant and grinned.

"Hey, sorry to butt in, but they're playing my favorite song and Mellie promised to dance it with me. Come on, sweetheart."

Spinning her around, he danced her away, using his hip to bump hers in time to the music, and her laughter was sweeter to him than chocolate fudge.

And he loved chocolate fudge.

"You realize you just said a thirty-year-old song about a donkey is your favorite, right?"

"Sure. Why not? I'm a vet, aren't I? And specifically known as an equine vet too. It's apt."

She was belly-laughing when they got to the dance floor and when he spun her, making that magical dress flare around her thighs, Delano realized he was lost.

Gone.

Destroyed by her beauty and sex appeal.

It should have scared him, this intense flare of

emotion, but somehow he just accepted it, deciding to contemplate what it meant at another time.

Right now, he was too busy enjoying her company, and her joy.

When the song finished, Mellie took his arm and steered him off the floor and back toward the table where the others sat.

"Thank you for the dance," she said demurely. "And for saving me from Martin. I thought he was going to take a bite out of my face, he was so close."

"I doubt he was thinking about biting. And I don't blame him. You're eminently kissable."

She stopped, her hand tightening on his arm, and turned a shining expression his way.

"If you feel that way, come home with me."

For a moment he couldn't move. Couldn't reply. His heart was thumping harder than the bass coming through the speakers, and an erotic rush almost took him to his knees.

Catching his breath took real effort, but as soon as he had he replied, "Gladly."

CHAPTER FOURTEEN

DELANO WASN'T SURE how Mellie wanted to handle
their departure. He didn't care if her friends knew
they were going home together, but there'd been
no time to discuss it with her before she'd started
walking again. The best he could do was let her
take the lead when they got back to the table.

Once there, she picked up her clutch and smiled
brightly at all their friends.

"Okay, folks. I'm heading home."

"Already?" Amity asked, looking at her watch.
"Oh, yeah. I know, I know. Early mornings…blah-
blah-blah."

"Not everyone can have a leisurely weekend like
you," Mellie rebutted, as she bent to hug her friend.
"My neighbors would be all over me like a cheap
suit if the animals started kicking up a fuss because
I hadn't fed them first thing."

The men all got up to say goodbye, and Delano
stood to one side, wondering if Mellie would give
him some kind of signal to show she meant what
she'd said.

Then he decided to take matters into his own
hands. After all, Mellie never said what she didn't
mean, at least as far as he'd seen to that point.

"Hey, do you mind giving me a ride home?" he

asked. "I came with Jason, but I promised Dad I'd help out around the house tomorrow, so I don't want to stay out too late."

"And you very much would be going home when the sun was up if you wait around for me," Jason said, with a chuckle. "Amity and I are known for being the last to leave parties like this."

"That's right, my brother from another mother," Amity said, getting up and pointing at the dance floor. "Let those old folks go home to bed, while we dance the night away."

And with one last wave they went off together, while Delano and Mellie started walking toward the car park.

"I'm parked about halfway down the driveway," she said, sounding a bit more subdued than she had earlier.

He hoped she wasn't having second thoughts, although he wouldn't blame her if she was. There was a part of him that wondered if sleeping with her was really a good idea—but that part wasn't strong enough to stop him from doing just that, if Mellie was still willing.

"I had a great time tonight." He didn't say it just to fill the silence between them, but because he really wanted her to know. "Your friends were great fun. But it was watching you enjoy yourself that really made it special."

She slanted him a glance. "I had a fabulous time too. I don't get out as much as I'd like to anymore, but work is more important."

"Is it?" They were approaching her vehicle, which was backed onto a strip of grass between two trees alongside the driveway, and she fished her keys out of her bag.

"Of course." She said it impatiently, as they left the dimly lit driveway, and entered the darker area beneath the trees. "What I do makes a difference—at least to the animals. I can't do it half-heartedly or let anything else get in the way."

"But what about you?" He reached for the handle to open the door for her, but paused. She was so near, and in the warmth of the night her scent wafted out to him, calling him closer. "Don't you deserve more than just work?"

"Deserve?" Mellie turned to him in the dark, and in the slight illumination coming from the party he saw the gleam of her eyes, and the sweet curve of her lips. "I don't think any of us deserve anything, except what we work for."

Just a step more, and their bodies would be almost touching.

Delano took that step.

"Have I worked hard enough to deserve a kiss?"

He heard her indrawn breath, then saw the flash of her teeth as she smiled.

"I believe you have."

Mellie leaned closer, leaving just a breath between their mouths, and Delano did what he'd been itching to all night. He ran one hand lightly down her side, over the silky fabric of her dress, from just below her breast until it came to rest on her hip. The experience didn't disappoint. In fact, it was even better than he'd imagined. The sensation of her curves beneath his fingers, the question of whether her skin would rival the smoothness of the material, almost undid him.

And feeling her shiver at his touch made waiting even one more second impossible.

He kissed her, but softly, holding back, teasing her lips with his, rubbing lightly back and forth, learning the contours of her mouth anew, inhaling each rushed breath as she exhaled. An electric charge fired between them, as though one of them was holding a live wire and the other one was grounded.

It was too much.

Not enough.

Not nearly enough.

When her tongue swept, soft and slick, across his lower lip, Delano's brain short-circuited.

The hand on her hip clenched to pull Mellie's body fully against his, his other hand going up to clasp her nape. She already had an arm around his neck and the other around his waist, clearly offering no resistance to either how tightly he held her nor the way he'd deepened their kiss.

Made it carnal and almost rough in his eagerness and need.

She turned so her back was against the car, pulling him with her, and he went willingly. They were fused, lips and torsos, her hand on his lower back, holding him as close as possible. Shifting slightly, he brought his knee up between her legs, settling her on his thigh, and she moaned low in her throat. He could feel the heat of her through his pants, and the sensation—coupled with all the others battering him—made him lose all sense of time and place.

Gripping her bottom, he pulled her a little higher and urged her to rock against him. He swallowed her next moan, and a gasp, and a truncated cry, as she sought her pleasure against his leg and he facilitated the hunt.

Mellie's head fell back against the car, breaking their kiss, and Delano took advantage of the motion to move his lips to her neck while his hand sought and found one breast. Beneath her bra her nipple was pebbled tight, and he pinched it and was flooded with savage satisfaction when she jerked and her movements became more frantic.

"Delano…" It was a whisper, wild and sweet. "I want… I need…"

"Let go," he said, his voice rough even to his own ears. "I have you, babe."

She grabbed his head, pulling it back up, and when their lips met again it was so he could absorb the sounds of her orgasm into his mouth, muffling the desire-struck moans and sighs of release.

Mellie came back down to earth, glad that Delano had her firmly in his embrace, since she wasn't sure her legs were even working. Resting her head against his shoulder, she attempted to catch her breath, enjoying the lingering echoes of her orgasm.

When last had she lost herself in passion that way? She couldn't remember. Wasn't even sure she ever had before.

Then the absurdity of the situation struck her befuddled brain, and she started to giggle.

Delano's arms tightened fractionally. "What?"

"I feel like a teenager again. Hiding in the shadows, making out. So horny all it takes is a well-positioned thigh to bring me off."

He was quiet for a moment, and then, as if he couldn't help it, he began to vibrate with suppressed laughter too. They'd been speaking in whispers, in case anyone else was around but, thankfully, Mellie saw no sign of onlookers.

What a view they would have had!

The thought made her giggle even harder, and she pressed her face into his shoulder to muffle the sound.

"Let's get out of here," Delano said, his voice a low growl, and Mellie became all too aware of his erection pressed against her belly.

The sensation brought another wave of arousal that made her shiver and killed her amusement.

"Yes." It came out rushed and a little harsh, and she took a deep breath before continuing, "I think my legs are working again."

He eased away, as though reluctant to let her go, and Mellie had to fight the urge to hang on to him.

Ridiculous to experience a sense of loss when he was still right there.

She stepped aside and reached for the door handle, but Delano's hand got there first.

"Such a gentleman," she said, laughing up at him.

"Seems incongruous to say, after what just happened," he rebutted, amusement rife in his tone.

"I don't know," she said in a demure tone, as she got into the driver's seat. "I was more than satisfied by your behavior."

He snorted, but when he bent into the car, bringing his face close to hers, there was no amusement evident in his expression.

"I hope to always bring satisfaction."

Before she could reply, he closed the door firmly and began to walk around to the passenger side. Just as well since her entire system had gone into overdrive at his words.

If he could achieve that, she'd be the happiest of women!

She started the car as he got in, and once they both had on their seat belts she backed out of the space beneath the trees and headed down the hill.

It was funny, but she didn't feel the need to fill the silence that had fallen between them. Usually, in a situation like this, which was still fraught with tension—albeit of the sexual kind—she'd chatter away, holding off any type of too-serious conversation. However, with Delano beside her, she didn't mind the quiet.

There was one thing she should speak to him about, though, before this went any further.

"You know that if you spend the night with me, your father will probably hear about it by sometime tomorrow. Port Michael is a hotbed of gossip, and whether I drop you home after a couple of hours, or you don't get home until morning, someone is sure to spill the beans."

"Unless someone saw us making out, at which point Aunt Eddie is getting a text right now." Mellie chuckled, but because she couldn't tell whether he was amused or rethinking their upcoming tryst, she didn't know how to respond. Luckily, Delano continued, "Does that bother you—that my father, and yours, would know we were together?"

"Not in a general sense," she replied, carefully. "I just don't want your dad to get the wrong idea. He's already hopeful that you'll come back here to live permanently, so if he thinks I'm an additional incentive for you to stay, it'll just make things worse for you."

"If that's all that's worrying you, put it out of your mind. I'll handle Dad if he asks me about us. Make it clear we're just enjoying ourselves, not getting serious."

"Okay." She made her reply as casual as his, but couldn't ignore the sudden pang of what felt like disappointment.

Not that she wanted him to be serious about her, right? The fact that Delano was only going to be around for a short time made him a safe, temporary partner. So why did it hurt to hear him say that?

Then she put that emotion aside.

After all, hadn't she once succumbed to the idea of everlasting love and happy-ever-after, and got burned by the delusion?

No. Being with Delano, who was hell-bent on going back to Trinidad as soon as possible, served her purpose well. Her long sexual drought would be over, but without strings and complications attached.

"What about your father?" His question made her glance over at him, but his face was too shadowed for her to see it. "Will I have Mr. Charlie coming after me to ask my intentions?"

"No." She said it decisively, very sure of the answer. "Daddy knows I can take care of myself."

He was the only one who knew exactly what she'd been through with Kyle. And that, thereafter, she was determined not to allow anyone to highjack her life or endanger her future.

Lesson learned!

"You know what's been driving me crazy all night?"

Delano's question jerked her out of her thoughts, and she was glad. They weren't what she wanted to be considering just now.

"What?"

"That dress you're wearing."

Again she tried to see his expression, but couldn't. She turned her attention back to the road, unable to stop herself from smiling. "Why?"

"It looks so soft, and it moves around you like

the definition of *temptation*. I was practically sitting on my hands in an effort not to touch you."

Mellie giggled. "If you're imagining some lacy undies beneath it, I'm going to have to disappoint you. The reason it moves the way it does is thanks to shapewear, which is anything but sexy."

"I'll be the judge of that," he growled in return, sending a rush of excitement over her skin to then arrow into her belly.

"I don't want you to be disappointed," she replied, but her voice quavered. She was still contemplating what else could happen once he got her underwear off.

She'd been fully clothed—shapewear included—when he'd given her an orgasm. Who knew what he was capable of when she had on less?

She'd taken the back way through the hills to her home, rather than go back into Port Michael proper, and as they approached her driveway Mellie's heart started thumping. She hit the button to open the gate. Once they'd driven inside, she closed it behind them and steered the car around to the back of the house, where she always parked.

Turning off the ignition, she said, "Do you mind closing the gate at the side of the house for me? That way I can let the dogs out of the house, but they'll be confined back here."

"Sure."

He got out of the vehicle before her and, as she locked the car, she watched him walk to the side of the house, enjoying the view. A shiver worked up her spine; the anticipation of what was about to happen made her legs tremble.

She waited for him by the back door, knowing the dogs would be startled to see him coming across the yard, and preferring to have him encounter them while he was with her.

When she opened the door, they dogs swarmed around them, but when she commanded them to go outside, they obeyed without a problem.

"They're well trained," he commented as he came up behind her. "They don't jump, and do as they're told, even though I'm sure they were looking at me sideways, wondering what I'm doing here at this time of night."

"I work at training them," she said, happy to be talking about something so mundane. "All the dogs that come here get some basic obedience instruction, either from me or from Johnny, but once I decide I'm keeping one, I do advanced training with them. With the number of animals they have to interact with, I can't afford to have any problems."

She heard the door close and the latch being turned as she waited in the dimness of the kitchen to lead him through to her bedroom. But after she'd taken just one step, Delano put his hand on her upper arm, bringing her to a halt.

"I can't wait," he whispered, coming up close behind her, his lips finding the tender flesh at the base of her neck, where it met her shoulder. "Let me touch you."

CHAPTER FIFTEEN

"COME THROUGH TO the bedroom." Mellie tried to keep her voice light, even amused, but it came out laden with desire all the same. "Isn't one teenage stunt enough for you tonight? The kitchen isn't the most comfortable place for lovemaking. At least, mine isn't."

His chuckle, rumbling into the skin of her nape, made her shiver.

"Perhaps you're right, but I don't want to let you go." His hands skimmed down her arms, leaving goose bumps in their wake, and then transferred to her hips, to skim up along her sides. "Your skin is even softer than this dress," he sighed.

"You're only letting me go for a minute." Grasping one of his hands, she led him through the house. "I promise, you won't be disappointed."

He didn't reply, but his fingers tightened on hers.

When they got to her bedroom door, Mellie turned the knob, commenting, "Slip in quickly. I don't want any of the cats in here tonight."

Delano chuckled. "Agreed," he said, and snugged up to her back, so they ended up going through the door practically fused together. As she giggled, it suddenly struck Mellie that she'd never enjoyed a sexual encounter as much as she was this one.

The undercurrents were heavy. The desire very real and arousing. But being able to laugh and tease and just be free with Delano was a new experience, and one she found remarkably appealing.

As soon as they were in her room, she turned on the light. He kicked the door closed behind them, and then there was no more time for laughter, because he'd spun her around and was kissing her.

No more hesitation or slow seduction now, but full-on passion that she returned wholeheartedly. Delano's hands skimmed her body as though trying to learn her shape, and when he tugged free the bow at her nape, which held her dress closed, he inhaled her gasp of acquiescence.

But when he began to gather the hem of her dress in preparation of taking it off over her head, she held on to the fabric and broke their kiss to tease, "Are you sure you're ready to be exposed to what I'm wearing underneath this?"

He was smiling, but the gleam in his eyes had nothing to do with amusement.

"I told you: I want to judge for myself whether it's alluring or not. You've whetted my interest with talking about this… What did you call it?"

"Shapewear."

"Yeah. The shapewear."

Still hanging on to the dress so he couldn't take it off without tearing it, she asked, "Surely you've seen it, or something similar, before?"

"Not that I'm aware of. At least, not on anyone,

in person. Now, will you let me see, before I explode with curiosity?"

Giggling again, she released her hold and raised her arms. Delano wasted no time in pulling the dress over her head, and Mellie kept her eyes closed for a long moment, letting her arms fall to her sides.

It was amusing, sure, but also a little embarrassing too. She hadn't really considered this part of the evening when she was getting dressed. If she had, she might have chosen a different outfit. One that could be worn with silk panties and a lacy bra. But all she'd thought of was how great the dress looked on, and what would best enhance the movement, which Delano had claimed to like so much.

Now here she was, trussed up a bit like a sausage in a high-waisted pair of shorts that went down to midthigh and a strapless boned long-line bra that met it, leaving not even a sliver of skin between.

She could hardly contain her laughter, as she cracked one eye open to find him examining her very closely indeed.

"Seductive, yeah?" she said, trying not to giggle-snort.

Those intent, gleaming eyes rose to hers, and quelled her amusement. But he didn't answer her question, either to agree or disagree.

Instead, he asked, "How on earth does this stay up?"

But she had to swallow a gasp when he accompanied the question with a sweep of one finger along the curve of the bra cups, skimming over the swell of her breasts rising above it. She licked her lips, which suddenly felt dry, as did her throat. Clearing it allowed her to speak.

"Are you really asking me to explain the physics of my underwear right now?"

"No." He circled her slowly, and when that inquisitive, arousing finger slid just below her bottom, outlining the lower curve, she realized for the first time just how sensitive those particular parts of her body were. "I'm actually trying to figure out the best way to get it all off."

"Should I give you a tutorial?" she asked. "Or just take it off myself?"

"No, no, no." There was something feral in his tone, and Mellie shivered to hear it. "That's definitely my job."

His hands explored—softly, but filled with determination. And she stood there, trembling, feeling each touch like a mini electric shock.

When he found the hidden zipper at the side of her bra, he made a sound of such satisfaction, goose bumps fired across her arms and back.

Nudging her arm out of the way, he found the tab with a deftness that surprised her, and pulled it down.

"You've done that before," she said, and although she'd wanted to make it sound accusatory and amused, her voice wouldn't cooperate.

"I'm a quick study." Oh, no mistaking the desire roughening the words as he gripped the bottom of the bra and she lifted her arms so he could free her from it.

Then he was standing in front of her, and something in his gaze made her want to cross her arms over her breasts. Not because it made her uncomfortable, but because the moment felt too raw and hot and real.

He growled a curse, his hand rising, his finger extended to circle her nipple, making it pull even tighter, sending a shockwave of pleasure through her body. There was no suppressing the moan that rose in her throat, and Delano echoed it.

Stepping closer, he dipped his head to pull the other nipple into his mouth, and Mellie arched, locking her knees so as not to melt into a puddle on the floor.

It took her a moment to realize Delano was, at the same time, working his hands into the sides of her shorts, stretching the elasticized fabric, pushing it inexorably down. When it got to her thighs, he released her nipple from his mouth and concentrated on getting the garment lower.

"I'm one of those people who likes taking my time to open my presents," he said, as he pushed the shorts down to her knees. "So I'm enjoying this immensely."

"That's a good thing." Mellie wanted to laugh, but her breathing was too erratic for that. In fact, it took real effort to get the words out past the lust tightening her throat. When he knelt at her feet, his face level with her stomach, she lost the ability to speak completely.

She could feel his breath against her skin, and the sensation made her belly flutter, the internal muscles rippling with desire.

Delano had unbuckled her sandals before she knew what he was about, and in an instant had both them and the shapewear shorts off. She expected him to rise, embrace her again, but he stayed where he was.

He traced a line across her thigh, where the elastic edge of the shorts had left an indentation. "This looks uncomfortable."

A wave of tenderness shook her, and she caressed his head, running her hand over the crisp, dark hair.

But she made her tone amused, as she said, "It's not painful. Just a small price to pay for fashion."

He looked up, and the expression in his eyes rocked her, although she didn't know exactly why.

"There's a price for every pleasure," he said.

Before she could figure out his meaning, or form a reply, he crouched farther and followed the path his finger had inscribed with his tongue.

"Oh!" Mellie gasped, her fingers tightening on his scalp.

Then he did it again, before switching to the other leg.

It shouldn't be an erogenous zone. It was the front of her thighs, only a few inches above her knees, but somehow those slick, sweet touches had her quaking with need.

Looking up at her again, Delano gripped her left ankle, urging her leg up. Unable to resist—not wanting to—she let him lift her leg and hook her knee over his shoulder. Then his hands came up to hold her bottom, and Mellie shuddered at being so securely held. Captured.

And he didn't break his gaze away from hers as he leaned forward and licked a line of what felt like erotic fire along the inside of her thigh.

Up, and up, that torturous tongue swept, stopping just short of where she so desperately wanted it to be, then reversing course to swirl and tease back toward her knee. The entire time he watched her face, and Mellie felt his attention like another touch.

Just as teasing.

Just as arousing.

Little nibbles now, along her thigh. Mobile lips sipping and tasting her skin, hinting at the variety of ways Delano was prepared to use that delicious mouth to bring her to completion.

She wanted to beg, to plead, but bit back the words. This was a new type of eroticism to her, and she found intense enjoyment in the anticipation. He was in no rush now. Not even for his own satisfaction.

Unlike most of the other men she's known, who'd have probably been finished and snoring by this point.

One hand still on his head, the other braced against the nearby wall, she let him have his way.

Gladly.

She was wholly unprepared for when his tongue finally swept through her folds, electrifying the already oversensitized flesh. Crying out in ecstasy, she fell forward, using his head and free shoulder as props to stop herself from falling, her body shuddering, yearning, reaching for the orgasm shimmering just beyond reach.

All Delano had promised with his lips and tongue on her thigh he delivered, and more. As she shook, and held his head in place, her hips rocking with a primal rhythm against his mouth, Mellie knew he was still teasing. Ratcheting her need higher with each skillful movement, keeping her hovering on the brink until, with a muffled shriek, she came.

But it was unlike any orgasm she'd had before. It continued, racking her, turning her inside out and rendering her insensate to everything but his mouth on her and the shocks firing out from that point to every inch of her body.

She was only vaguely aware of Delano standing, somehow keeping her on her feet until he could pick her up and carry her to the bed.

The coverlet under her skin was cool, and somewhat soothing, but couldn't quench her excitement. Forcing her eyes open, she was in time to see Delano toss his wallet onto the bedside table. He unfastened only the top two buttons of his shirt before pulling it off over his head, his rush to undress completely in line with her eagerness to see him naked.

How could it be, she wondered, that after that incredible orgasm, she still was aroused and wanting him in the most intimate way possible?

She thought about sitting up and helping him get his pants off, but besides her limbs feeling like overcooked spaghetti, she was enjoying the view too much from where she was.

Rippling muscles across his chest and abdomen. Not the kind gained at a gym, but from working with the horses, probably, and his propensity for running each morning. Then he was bending to push his pants down, and Mellie lost her ability to breathe, even before he'd straightened.

Gorgeous.

She would have told him that was what she thought, but he had lowered himself onto the bed and was gathering her close, and she realized she'd rather kiss him than speak.

But she could let her hands and lips do the talking.

Delano felt as though he was about to vibrate right out of his skin.

Being with Mellie was everything he'd dreamed it would be, and so much more.

It wasn't just that she was passionate and so responsive it blew his mind. There was something else between them that took his desire for her to a whole new level.

And despite not being sure what that something was, he just wanted to revel in it.

In her.

She'd twined her arms and one leg around him as they lay face-to-face on the bed, and although he was so aroused it hurt, Delano felt no urge to stop kissing her. Instead, what he wanted was to bring her to orgasm one more time, because watching and hearing her achieve bliss had been the biggest turn-on of his life.

But Mellie was running her hands all over his body, fingers smoothing and squeezing his arms and back and thighs, and the sensation was sublime. It was as if she wasn't just learning his body, but admiring it at the same time. It was probably just his ego speaking, but that didn't stop him from feeling amazed and amazing.

Before he lost his mind completely to passion, still intent on pleasuring her again, he reached down and hiked her leg higher so it rested almost at his waist. Then he snaked his hand over her thigh and found the wetness between her legs.

"Delano!" She pulled back to gasp.

"Do you want me to stop?" He kept his fingers poised at her opening, but still gave her the option to say yes or no.

"No," she moaned, as though the word hurt to utter. "Definitely don't stop."

Elated, he bent to kiss and suck along her throat, and was rewarded when she arched, bringing her hips closer while baring her neck to his marauding mouth.

She was panting, little moans of delight breaking from those luscious lips. The heat between them intensified, and her inner muscles tightened around his fingers, making him groan in turn. She was so tight and wet and hot, he was sure being inside her intimately would be better than any other sexual experience he'd ever had before.

Suddenly she rolled, pushing him onto his back, breaking free from his hand and lips and grasp. When she leaned over him, she was more beautiful in that moment than he could bear. Her lips soft and swollen, her cheeks flushed, eyes dark with desire and gleaming. Rumpled and needy and determined.

And his.

"Condom."

She didn't ask a question but made a demand, and, without breaking eye contact, he reached back over his head to where he'd tossed his wallet. Mellie leaned over him to get it, and he took advantage of the motion to pull a succulent nipple between his lips. Her little mewl did nothing to dissuade, but after a moment she sat back, and he had to let it go.

She'd found the prophylactic, and tore the packet open carefully.

"I can do it," he said, his voice like gravel with the force of his need.

Mellie just smiled, and palmed his erection. When she stroked it from base to tip and back again, his hips lifted of their own accord, and heat gathered in the small of his back.

"Mmm…" she hummed, having her way with him, even when he gave a pleading groan. "No. I'll take care of it."

It was, he thought hazily, payback of the sweetest sort. If she'd asked, he'd have admitted to teasing her, wanting to give her pleasure that stretched and soared before reaching the final crescendo. But she didn't ask, and he knew she didn't need to, because she'd already sussed him out and didn't hesitate to repay him in kind.

All her movements were slow, and sure. Stroking, squeezing, caressing, until Delano closed his eyes as tightly as possible, hoping the star-shot darkness would help him maintain some semblance of control.

Yet, he wouldn't stop her, even when he felt he had to, or risk coming at a time, and in a way, he least wanted to. It was more important to cede the control to her right now than it was to try to snatch it back.

As though knowing the exact moment she had pushed him just shy of his limit, Mellie ceased her torture and smoothly rolled on the condom.

That, in itself, was almost too much for Delano, who clenched his jaw hard against the sensation. At least the tightening of the sheath around the base of his erection quelled some of his urge to orgasm, but only a little.

Before he could move, Mellie straddled his thighs, and the breath left his throat in a rush.

"Wait," he said, so dazzled by the desire in her eyes he knew he'd be lost as soon as she took him into her body. "Give me a minute."

She smiled and nodded, but her fingers danced over his hips to his belly, and stroked across his abs.

"You know, you're really quite beautiful without your clothes."

Her words surprised a bark of laughter from him.

"So, I'm ugly with them on?"

Mellie wrinkled her nose. "Now you're just fishing for compliments. But seriously, some people look amazing when they're dressed, but not so hot naked. You, however, look fabulous whether clothed or not." She tilted her head, as though considering her own words. "I think it has something to do with the way you carry yourself—although the muscles don't hurt either."

Silly to be awash with pride. Especially since he didn't place much store in good looks, either in himself or others. But it was impossible not to be pleased with the knowledge that Mellie found him attractive, although if she hadn't, he doubted they'd be where they were right now.

And the conversation had given him the breathing room he needed, tempering his arousal just enough that he believed he wouldn't embarrass himself like a schoolboy having his first sexual experience.

Sitting up, he wrapped his arms around Mellie's

waist and she leaned in to kiss him. The passion between them flared white-hot again, and she lifted gracefully in his embrace, positioning herself, and then lowering to take him in all at once.

They both froze, panting, and Delano thought his heart would pound out of his chest at the sublime sensation.

"Oh," she gasped, as if having made a shocking discovery.

Then she captured his lips again, and began to move. Flowing, rocking, rising, falling, as he held and touched and kissed her, never wanting to stop. Never wanting this feeling of pleasure and belonging and happiness to end.

When the end came, as it had to, Delano had no control over it because it was the sight and sound and feel of Mellie's orgasm that threw him over the edge and sent him into the stratosphere.

CHAPTER SIXTEEN

DELANO AWOKE TO a light weight on his chest, and an unmistakable sound humming in his ears. When he opened his eyes, it was to meet the green-gold gaze of the black kitten, who was happily making biscuits in the covers draped over Delano's torso and purring like crazy. Weak predawn sunlight came in through a chink in the curtains and semi-open bedroom door.

"Gilligan." Mellie's voice came from the doorway, and Delano turned to watch her walk in, searching her expression for her reaction to their night together. She looked calm and cool, and was already dressed, which made him conscious of the fact he was completely naked beneath the sheet. "How did you get in here? You're a menace and a real escape artist."

"But you love him," Delano said, hearing the fondness in her tone, and lifting said menace so he could sit up.

Mellie smiled ruefully. "I do. I think he might be a foster fail. If I were a witch, I'd have him as my familiar. He's so full of personality and life." Then she sent Delano a mischievous glance, as she held out a cup of coffee to him. "But he seems to love you even more than me. Maybe you should have him."

"Oh, I don't think so. Baldur is great with other animals, even cats, but something tells me there may be a jealous streak in Gilligan."

"Maybe," she said, brushing her hands down the legs of her jeans. "And I'm guessing Baldur sees you as his, alone?"

"I'm not sure how he'd feel about sharing his space with another animal. It's been just the two of us living together since I got him. My older dog had died just a short time before."

Mellie sat carefully on the edge of the bed so as not to joggle his hand and spill the coffee. Strange, and yet heartening, to have such a commonplace conversation after a night of spectacular sex!

"I think you're the only vet I know who doesn't have a houseful of animals. Well, at least three or four."

He blew on the hot liquid and took a cautious sip before replying. "You know I was married, right?" She nodded, so he went on, "My ex didn't like animals, but still married a vet. Go figure. She would only agree to us having one dog—no cats, she couldn't stand them—because she said any more than that would make too much of a mess in the house. I just kind of got used to it."

Her snort was slightly derisive, but more amused than anything else.

"You should have brought one of the horses home instead of a dog."

He couldn't help laughing at that, and when Mellie leaned forward and kissed him lightly, it felt so natural he was taken aback.

She didn't give him time to reply, or even to deal with whatever the strange emotion washing through him was.

Picking up Gilligan, she stood and said, "Drink your coffee and get dressed so I can take you home and get back here to deal with the animals."

"I could help."

She shook her head, grinning, as she headed for the door, the kitten held firmly in her grasp.

"Not in your party clothes. You're better off doing the walk of shame back at your dad's at sunrise than turning up later in the day looking like you went through a hedge backward."

She was right, of course, but Delano couldn't help feeling let down. Like it was an anticlimax after what they'd shared the night before.

The truth was, he realized as he took a quick shower in her neat and tidily arranged bathroom, he didn't want to leave.

Okay. Didn't want to leave Mellie.

He'd enjoyed himself last night, even more than he'd thought he would. Sure, the sex had been off-the-charts hot, but it was more than that. Mellie herself had made it special. With her laughter, wry humor, playfulness and passion.

It had been an experience unlike any other, and he didn't want it to end.

He would have liked to spend the day with her,

carrying on the conversations, sharing the laughter, and, yes, tumbling her back into bed and making her cry out with ecstasy.

But he really had promised his father to take care of some things around the house. That hadn't just been a line to excuse his leaving the party with Mellie the night before. So, although he regretted the necessity, he really did have to go back to Dad's.

Besides, it was too soon to have everyone know he and Mellie were having—

What were they having, exactly?

Sex only?

A friends-with-benefits-type thing?

A fling?

None of those seemed quite right but, as Delano dried off, he couldn't find the proper description.

Not that he should be trying to categorize it, anyway. In a couple of weeks, at the most, he'd be gone. Back to Trinidad, and his comfortable, normal life.

Giving their relationship a title would just make things more complicated.

"Hey, how're you getting on in there?" she called, as he was pulling on his shirt.

Man, she was eager to get rid of him!

"Just coming." He shoved his feet into his shoes, a little annoyed now, but more with himself than with Mellie. They'd both known this wasn't the beginning of a love affair, but here he was, acting like she'd promised more than she was willing to deliver.

When he went into the living room, she was coming back in from the attached cattery.

"The last of the older kittens will be going off to their new homes today, so I can put Gilligan and his sisters in the nursery, and get back my powder room," she said.

"Unless you have more kittens come in," he said, half teasing, half serious.

She snorted, and shook her head. "Or a pregnant bitch. My whelping boxes are full too. If you're ready, I'll just grab my bag and keys, and we can go."

"Sure."

He'd taken his cup into the kitchen, and by the time he'd washed it and put it to drain, she was standing by the back door, ready to leave.

"You're well trained," she said, using her chin to point to the sink.

"Aunt Eddie raised me to be able to take care of myself," he admitted. "Her advice has always been *Never be a burden to anyone, or let a woman tie you by your stomach.*"

"What did she mean by that?" Mellie asked, obviously amused. She unlocked the car as they got near to it, and Delano realized the side gate was already open. "I don't think I've ever heard that expression before."

"Just that I should learn to cook, and do whatever I needed to do to live comfortably by myself." He opened the car door and then slid in, as Mellie did the same on the other side. "Some of the older generation of men were so used to being catered to, she was determined I wasn't going to be like them."

"Makes sense. And good for her."

As Mellie started the car, there was a cacophony of barks from the kennel building, and the dogs started streaming out. Johnny Luck must be up and letting them all out, and Delano was reminded of what Amity had told him the night before, about the fact that the shelter was at capacity.

It worried him, for a couple of reasons.

Mellie wanted to buy his father out and take over the clinic, but she also needed to expand the shelter. From what Aunt Eddie had said, and Amity intimated, Mellie couldn't afford to do both.

If that was the case, and the shelter was at capacity, would she be tempted to prioritize the shelter over the clinic, when it came time to decide where to spend her money?

Although Delano had no interest in taking over the clinic himself—since it meant staying in St. Eustace—he'd feel sad and guilty if his father had no choice but sell it to someone else. There were other vets in Port Michael who'd probably be happy to buy out the practice, and take Mellie on as an associate. But he knew both Mellie and his father really wanted it to go to her.

"You're very quiet."

Mellie's voice pulled him out of his ruminations. She seemed to be trying to sound casual, but there was no mistaking the question in her tone.

"Woolgathering, and still a little bit sleepy," he

replied, intercepting a sideways glance from her as he turned to look her way. "Can you blame me, after such a fabulous night?"

Her lips turned up in a sly smile that made him want her all over again.

"It was rather nice, wasn't it?"

"Nice?" He didn't have to feign his outrage. "Nice?"

Mellie giggled, her cheeks darkening with a blush. "Very, very nice, indeed."

"Well, I'm going to have to try harder next time, aren't I? How about tonight?"

"I think that will work. Come by whenever you're free."

Yet, he realized he was reluctant to part from her, and the only sop to his longing was the sweet, lingering kiss she gave him before he got out of the car.

"See you later," she said, with a little wave.

And Delano watched her back out of the driveway, discontentment chasing away much of his lingering pleasure.

Mellie spent the day working at the shelter, and grinning.

A lot.

She found herself swinging from elation at the night just gone and surprise that no one called to ask what she thought she was doing, having Delano overnight at her house. It never occurred to her that it might still not be common knowledge, nor to consider not having him over later.

No use quibbling over how Delano had made her feel.

Beautiful.

Desirable.

More than enough.

The last thought brought her up a little short, and she rested on the rake she was using to clean the fowl coop for a moment, considering it.

In hindsight she could see the way Kyle had gaslit her into thinking there was something not quite enough about her for him. Even when he was using her, he'd subtly complained about all she was doing, and even about her attractiveness. He'd come home in the evenings, after she'd spent the day working on the house, nitpick at what she'd done and sniff at her clothes.

As though he'd expected her to be dressed in a ballgown after putting in baseboards, hanging crown molding or painting all day. And when she'd said she was tired, he had no qualms about going out without her, and telling her she was getting boring.

He'd hoped, of course, she'd be so dispirited by it that when he'd ultimately betrayed her, she'd be inclined to take the blame on herself. In fact, knowing about her fraught relationship with her mother, who expected everyone else to accept responsibility when things went wrong, he'd anticipated it.

Mellie shook her head sharply, and went on with

her raking. Although at the time she hadn't fully evolved out of the doormat mentality she'd grown up with, she was well on the way. And she'd made sure Kyle hadn't got away with what he'd done.

Coming out on the other side of that contretemps, bloodied but unbowed, vindicated and determined never to be lied to and used that way again, had been one of her life's highlights. The final step on her path to true, independent adulthood.

Happiness came with finding her place, here in St. Eustace. In seeing a need beyond her work, which was satisfying in itself, and filling it as best she could. She didn't try to fool herself into thinking she'd always be able to manage both the practice and the shelter. Rescue in itself could easily become a full-time job, which was why she'd sought advice and set it up as a not-for-profit, with a board of directors she could depend on to help the shelter grow.

No, it was all worked out; or it would be, once Dr. Milo made up his mind what he wanted to do.

It was a shame that Delano didn't want to come back and live on the island of his birth, but he seemed adamant. Unlike his father, Mellie could only respect his choice, although she speculated about it. Being a racecourse vet and even an associate in someone else's clinic wasn't the same as having your own establishment.

It made her wonder what the real reason was for his refusal to come home.

Then she reminded herself that it was none of

her business, no matter how curious she was. There was an agreement between her and Delano, tacit, if not specifically spelled out, that there would be no emotional attachment. And even if she found herself mooning over just how fabulous he was in bed, and how much she enjoyed his company outside of it, she'd do well not to pry.

Finished with her chores, she put away her rake and headed to the cottage, pushing all the weighty thoughts aside and turning her attention to a very important question: What was she going to wear tonight, besides her favorite peacock blue lace undies?

Or should she bother to wear anything over them at all?

Just the thought was enough to make her laugh, and cause a frantic wash of lust through her system.

Yes. She liked that idea a lot.

And was sure Delano would too.

CHAPTER SEVENTEEN

SOMETIME—AND SHE wasn't exactly sure when—
Mellie had decided to simply enjoy Delano while
she could. And she'd been glad of that choice after
talking to him later in the evening.

He'd been honest about his intention to go back
to Trinidad as soon as he could. Looked at from
that perspective—that maybe she had as little as a
week with him—Mellie could relax and just enjoy
their time together.

And she did enjoy him, to the fullest. Delano
was the most selfless and attentive lover she'd ever
had. Waking up each morning, filled with memories of the night before, had her smiling and in the
best of moods.

If there were any clouds in her blue-sky attitude,
they manifested whenever she actually allowed herself to think about what her life would be once he
was gone.

The truth was that he'd become more than a lover
to her, and although she staunchly refused to give
a name how she felt, it was useless to deny she
would miss him.

Terribly.

She'd forgotten how it felt to be with someone
who not only stimulated her sexuality but also her

mind. They could talk about almost anything, laugh together, work together. She'd taken to sharing her thoughts and plans with him, without reservation. Telling herself she felt that free and comfortable with him because she knew he wouldn't be around much longer became a refrain she wished she fully believed.

On the Wednesday before the spay and neuter clinic, Delano came into the office at lunchtime, Baldur at his heels.

"Hey," he said, coming to lean against her desk. "I had an idea I wanted to pass by you. Have you considered arranging a freedom flight for some of your animals? Sending them to the US or Canada to be adopted?"

Mellie rocked back in her chair, and nodded slowly.

"I have, but I don't have any contacts abroad to make it happen."

His grin made goose bumps fire out across her chest, and tightened her nipples.

The man was too damned sexy for his own good—and hers!

"I do. My friend Sam Nichols runs the Vaughn Shelter just outside of Toronto. I've known her and her brother for years, and I called her and asked her advice. She's thrilled by the opportunity to help."

Mellie sat back, staring at him. It was, on the surface, a great idea. A shelter in Jamaica had done something similar in the past, sending over a hundred dogs to Canada and new homes. If they could pull it off, it really would give them some breathing space. However, to Mellie, there was the other side of the equation.

Delano hadn't asked if this was something Mellie would consider. He'd just gone ahead and reached out to his Canadian friend.

It smacked of him sidelining her, despite the fact that the shelter was *hers*.

"What's wrong?" Delano's eyebrows dipped into a frown, and he tipped his head to the side, as though trying to figure out why she wasn't over the moon about it.

"Nothing," she said quickly, not wanting to sour his pleasure at what he'd done, although at the moment she couldn't share it. "How do I contact your friend Sam?"

"I gave her your number, and she said she'd call you." He was still eyeing her narrowly. "Are you sure you're okay?"

It was the perfect opening to express her annoyance, but she didn't take it, needing time to figure out why she'd had that knee-jerk reaction. Putting it aside for the moment, she smiled and, instead, asking if he was ready for obedience class that evening.

"As ready as I can be. Dad is coming with me, so I better bring my A game."

"He's not that much of a stickler." Mellie jumped to Dr. Milo's defense. "Also, he'll probably be so happy to get out of the house, he won't care if the entire class is a shambles."

Delano chuckled in agreement. "That's probably true. Dad's not used to being stuck at home like this with Aunt Eddie hovering over him and making him rest—not if all the chores he's given me since I arrived are any indication."

"Very true. Your father has slowed down a bit over the last couple of years, but was still one of the busiest men I know."

Delano was slowly stroking his hand along her neck, from just beneath her ear to her shoulder, giving her goose bumps. Not that she minded.

"Do you have time to have dinner with me this evening, before obedience class? Then we could go together. Dad's been asking for you."

That was something she really liked about him. He never demanded her time, but always asked if she was available. In the past she would have been quite content to say no, citing work at the shelter, but she was already considering how best to accommodate him.

"I think so."

"Great." Bending, he placed a lingering kiss on her lips, before getting to his feet. "By the way, what time should I be ready to go to the spay and neuter clinic on Saturday?"

It was an opportunity to ask when he was planning to go back to Trinidad, but Mellie let it pass, wanting to know and yet not wanting to, as well. She was just glad he was actually sticking around, at least until then.

"It's about an hour to Grand Harbor, depending

on the traffic, and I usually try to get to the venue by about seven thirty to set up and help with registration if necessary."

"I'll be ready then." He paused, halfway to the door, and continued, "If I'm not already with you."

She was smiling to herself as he went out the door. If she had anything to say about it, they definitely would be together on Saturday morning. Then the smile faded, to be replaced with a wave of melancholy. By then she suspected they'd be on a countdown to his departure, and she wanted to spend as much time with him as possible.

Unfortunately, she had to cancel their dinner plans that evening, and tell him she'd probably miss obedience class.

"Your friend Sam contacted me and wants to teleconference tonight to start making plans." Mellie had forgiven Delano about the freedom flight too, knowing she was being unreasonable. His excitement about possibly helping the shelter had been palpable. "The board and I will be talking to her about what we need to do to get it off the ground."

"Okay. I'll miss you at obedience class, but that's more important. Can I come by your place afterward?"

They were alone in the office, the last patients for the day seen and the staff already gone. Mellie couldn't resist moving into his arms and kissing Delano, reveling in the surge of desire that immediately swamped her.

"Of course," she finally replied, a little breath-lessly, when they finally parted. "I'd be very disap-pointed if you didn't."

Obedience class went better than Delano expected, mainly because most of the lookie-loos from the week before didn't bother to come back. And when everyone saw his father walking in, the jubilation was unmistakable. A good half an hour went by, with everyone crowding around him in the pavil-ion, before Delano could get the class started.

"Where's Mellie?" Kiah Langdon asked, just as Delano was getting everyone situated.

"She had some business to take care of this eve-ning," he replied, hoping no one noticed the disap-pointment in his voice.

His father had been disappointed too, when told Mellie probably wouldn't make it. Although they spoke on the phone almost every day, she hadn't been by the house since Delano had arrived.

"You tell Mellie I want to see her, okay?" Dad said, as Delano was in the process of dropping him back off at home after the class.

It was the only time his father had intimated he knew where Delano was spending his evenings, and nights.

"I will, Dad," he replied, half expecting for his father to segue into a more detailed line of ques-tioning about the relationship between his son and his associate, but nothing more was said. Maybe just knowing Delano was going back to Trinidad soon was enough to make him hold his tongue.

When he got to Mellie's it was to find her in a state of cautious excitement.

"Sam was very helpful, and we have a tentative action plan in place," Mellie told him as she paced back and forth across her living room, the dogs' heads following her movements as if they were watching a tennis match. "Next week, we're going to start picking the dogs we think will do best, and photographing them, sourcing kennels—although Sam thinks she can help with that—and speaking to the government vet. Luckily, I know him well, and can count on his discretion. We're going to keep this as quiet as we can, until we know whether we can bring it off or not."

"Have you thought about contacting the shelter in Jamaica and asking how they managed?"

Mellie shook her head. "Sam is speaking to one of the people who was involved in that freedom flight, and they're advising her how best to go about it." She paused then, and turned her gleaming gaze his way, and something in that look made his heart gallop. "Have I properly thanked you for this?"

"Sure," he replied, as she stalked closer to where he was sitting on the couch.

"I'm pretty sure I haven't," she said. "I was annoyed about it at first because you didn't ask me before contacting Sam."

The shock of her words had him sitting up, horrified.

"Why didn't you say something, Mel, so I could apologize? I didn't mean for it to look like I was doing an end run around you, or something. I was just so excited by the idea, I went ahead with it."

She smiled then, shaking her head.

"It was a knee-jerk reaction." She seemed to consider for a moment, before lowering herself into a chair so she was facing him across the coffee table. Was it intentional that she kept a distance between them? "I have a problem with anything that seems to threaten my autonomy. I'm not very trusting, as you know all too well."

He wasn't sure if she'd answer, but it seemed important to ask, "Is there a particular reason?"

"A couple." Her brow wrinkled, as though she was wondering why they were talking about it, but then she gave a small shrug and continued, "I told you a little about my mother, and her reaction to my contacting Daddy."

"Yes." Something held him still, poised at the edge of his seat, surprised she was opening up to him in this way.

"Well, that was the final break, but the rift between us had been growing for a long time. All my life she's been demanding, wanting me to do whatever she said, without question. But as I got older, I realized she also lied, a lot, to get her way. When you're a child, and realize you can't depend on your parent to be truthful, you stop trusting everyone."

She took a deep breath and shook her head.

"She didn't want me to be a vet. She told me she and my stepfather couldn't afford my tuition. I took out loans and worked to get through vet school, only to find out afterward that Daddy had been sending her my college fees. When we figured it out, he made her give me the money so I could pay off the rest of my loans, but that sense of betrayal intensified."

Delano wanted to go to her. Hold her. But everything about her posture told him it would be the wrong thing to do just then.

So all he said instead was, "I'm sorry, Mel."

The movement of her lips might have been an attempt at a smile, but it didn't succeed.

"You'd think I'd have learned my lesson, wouldn't you? But I didn't. I was engaged to a man who treated me almost the exact same way. He isolated me from my friends by getting me to move to Miami with him, took my savings as a down payment on a house, used me to help fix it up, then sold it out from under me. Kyle kicked me out on Christmas Eve, leaving me with almost nothing."

Now she smiled, a ferocious grin that eased the anger welling inside him.

"But he'd underestimated me, you know? He knew what I'd gone through with Mom, and figured I'd be too embarrassed or weak to do anything about it, but I'd learned from Daddy that you don't let people get away with things like that. The money I have put away is what I won when I sued him for both my savings and punitive damages."

He couldn't bear it anymore. Delano got up and strode around the intervening table, Mellie's gaze following his movements. When he reached her, he opened his arms, his heart thundering in his ears, as he waited to see if she'd accept his offer of comfort and solace.

When she did, rising to step into his arms, Delano closed his eyes, more thankful than he could express, even to himself.

"Oh, sweetheart," he said, when he'd gotten control of his anger, sorrow and voice. "I'll never lie to you, ever. And now that I know how you feel, I'll always ask your opinion before I interfere in your business."

Mellie didn't answer, except to pull his head down and kiss him. Not passionately. At least, not at first. Instead, it felt like a promise, as well as an act of forgiveness and understanding.

But it didn't take long for the desire that always flowered when they were together to rise into a flame, and then a conflagration that wouldn't be quenched without the ultimate intimacy. And Delano didn't resist when she led him to her bedroom, although a part of him whispered that they'd crossed a dangerous line, and there could be no going back.

Even if he'd wanted to retreat.

CHAPTER EIGHTEEN

THE NEWS OF the commission's findings in the racing scandal was in the newspaper that Friday morning, and Delano was reminded, once again, that he should be booking his flight back to Trinidad.

His father was doing well. The doctor had assured Delano that in a week or so Milo would be cleared to resume working, although he was advised to slow down somewhat.

"You're not getting any younger, Milo," Dr. Fleetwood had said. "And I think this infarction was a shot across your bow. A warning you'd be wise to heed."

There'd been some grumbling from Dad, but resignation too.

In fact, Delano thought his father was looking forward to turning more of the clinic matters over to Mellie.

"I don't think I'm ready to retire fully," he'd said, when Delano was driving him back to the house after his appointment. "These past weeks have been too quiet for me. But it was also nice not to be rushing around and worrying about everything."

"Mellie kept everything running smoothly the whole time. Once you decide what you want to do, I'm sure she'll be willing to discuss it with you."

His father had only grunted in reply, and Delano hadn't pushed for anything more.

Their relationship had definitely improved over the time he'd been back in St. Eustace, and Delano didn't want to do anything to jeopardize it. Taking Mellie's advice to start from where they were, and look to the future rather than the past, had proven to be the right course.

They hadn't spoken much about his mother, but it was a start. Delano knew he would never get over his guilt, and his father might never fully recover from his son's part in his wife's death, but they could make the most of the time they had left.

Perhaps that was why each time he thought of booking his ticket, Delano found something else to occupy his time, or an excuse for waiting?

Yet, even as he thought it, he knew he was lying to himself.

It was Mellie keeping him on St. Eustace.

But he was set on returning to Trinidad, and his life there. The haunting recollections had faded, but he knew it was just temporary. The weight of his responsibility never left him, had only abated in the face of the passionate relationship he had with Mellie.

The clinic was busy, and they'd already agreed that he would finish up the last of the clients that evening, while Mellie prepped for the spay and neuter clinic the following day. At about two thirty, she came into the examination room, as soon as the patient he'd been with left.

"Okay," she said, looking down at the list in her hand. "I think I have everything, and whatever is forgotten I can take with us tomorrow. I'm heading out to Grand Harbor with this load."

"What time will you be back?"

She shrugged. "Not before about five. Probably a little later. We could have dinner, if you're free."

"Sounds good. Drive safely."

The exam room door was open, so he didn't try to kiss her goodbye. Although everyone at the clinic probably knew they were sleeping together, they did their best not to flaunt it.

But as he watched her bustle out, he wished he'd had the chance.

Soon those sweet salutes would be a thing of the past.

It hurt to think that, and he was honest enough to know it was because he'd fallen for Mellie. Not far enough to overcome his antipathy toward the island of his birth and all the painful memories that resided here, but enough that the thought of leaving her was a wrench.

He wouldn't express his feelings to her, especially not after hearing all she'd been through. She had good reason not to trust when she'd been so horribly treated. To confess he was more than halfway in love with her, but wouldn't do anything concrete about it, would sound a likely story.

He'd considered asking her if she'd consent to a long-distance affair, with one or the other of them traveling back and forth, but knew that made no sense. Mellie's life was full. Between the clinic and the shelter, she had no time for flying to Trinidad to see him, and once his father retired, or semiretired, she'd be even busier.

It wouldn't be possible for him to fly back regularly either. Races were run at the track twice a week, and he worked three or four days at the vet clinic where he was employed. When could they ever coordinate with schedules like that?

No.

A clean break was what would suit them both.

Besides, Mellie had given no indication of wanting him to stay, or to extend their affair. He liked to think they could sustain the friendship that had grown between them, but there was no room for any further development of their relationship.

A depressing thought, but the truth nonetheless.

There was one patient left to be seen for the day, and Delano was prepping the exam room when the door flew open and Leila, the vet tech, rushed in, holding a pet carrier.

"Wounded cat," she said. "The owner says dogs got at it."

A teenage boy came in behind her, the fear and distress on his face unmistakable.

"He's an indoor/outdoor cat, but he usually stays in our yard," he babbled, as Delano and Leila put on their gloves. "I don't know why he went down the road and into the neighbor's yard."

Looking into the carrier, Delano could see one of the cat's eyes was swollen shut, and blood matted the fur around its neck and flank. The animal looked to be in shock, and hissed as soon as it saw Delano's face through the door.

"Get the bite-proof gloves," he said over his shoulder to Leila. Then he sent the young man a questioning glance. "What's your cat's name?"

"Hero," he replied, his voice cracking a little on the word.

"And yours?"

"Marcus."

"Okay, Marcus." Delano kept his voice calm and reassuring. "We're going to take the top off the carrier, and make sure he doesn't try to run away, but I can see he's in a lot of pain, so Hero will probably fight us. If you're up for it, will you stay and try to calm him down by speaking to him? If he hears a familiar voice, it might help."

"Sure," the teen said, trying to sound confident, but his voice wavered.

Hero was traumatized and, from his attempts to bite and scratch, just wanted to be left alone, but they were able to get him out of the carrier and subdued on the table long enough to be sedated. Once he was asleep, Delano examined him, while Leila began cleaning him up, looking for any missed puncture marks or wounds as she went.

"Hero has a number of bite marks," Delano told Marcus, "but they're not from dogs. If it had been dogs that had attacked him, the bites would be bigger, and deeper." And the cat probably wouldn't have survived, but he didn't add that part. "It looks as though he was fighting with another cat. How old is he?"

"Umm…" Marcus seemed to be doing sums in his head before he said, "Just about a year old, I think."

And still intact. That would explain a lot. He'd probably strayed into an older tom's domain, on the trail of a female, and gotten into a fight.

"He's reached sexual maturity," Delano explained. "And that means he's going to start going after females. The only way to stop that from happening is to get him neutered."

"I thought about doing that, but it's real expensive, and my mam won't pay for it."

Delano was stitching up the worst of Hero's cuts, and Marcus was gently stroking one of the now-still paws. It was clear that the youngster really cared for his cat, and was worried.

"Dr. Mellie, who also works here, runs spay and neuter clinics," he told the young man. "They do it at low or no cost. Unfortunately, the next one is tomorrow, and Hero is too hurt to have surgery right now. But if you keep checking, I'm sure there'll be another one soon."

"I think I heard Dr. Mellie say they're planning one in three or four weeks, right here," Leila added. "Hopefully Hero will be well enough then, but you'll have to bring him and let Dr. Mellie look at him to make sure."

Delano felt a pang, like loss, at the thought that by then he'd be long gone. He still hadn't made a decision on when he was leaving, but he knew it would have to be soon. The longer he stayed, the harder it would be for him to leave.

They patched Hero up, and Delano told Marcus he'd like to keep the cat in the hospital for a couple of days.

"Unless you think you'll be able to put the medicine in his eye yourself?"

The teen looked doubtful. "I don't know if he'll let me. He scratched me up good when I was putting him in the carrier, and he's usually good about that."

So it was arranged that Hero would stay at the clinic over the weekend, and Marcus left to go home and treat his own wounds.

"Did the last client stay?" Delano asked Leila when she came back into the room from putting Hero in a cage down in the hospital.

"She did. Her dog's just here for boosters, worming and a wellness check."

"Thank goodness," Delano said with a chuckle. It was almost five o'clock, and the appointment had been for four. "When you send her in, you can go on home. It doesn't make sense for both of us to be late."

"Thanks, Doc." Leila grinned as she sanitized the examination table. "No word of a lie, but I'm starving."

He was just finishing his notes when he heard the door behind him open, and a voice he hadn't heard in over twenty years said quietly, "Delano?"

He froze, his brain seizing for an instant. An icy wave rushed through his body, and when he turned to face the woman behind him, it was with the stiff, jerky movements of a much older man.

"Mrs. Gopaul?"

She smiled, but Delano didn't think it got all the way to her eyes.

"It's good to see you, Del," said his friend Everard's mother. "It's been a very long time."

Mellie left Grand Harbor to head back to Port Michael, her head full of lists and plans for the following day. At some point in the future, what she really wanted was to buy a mobile veterinarian clinic, or make one, if necessary. An old RV would work, and that way she could go into the nooks and crannies of the island, instead of having to find a clinic where the spay and neuter events could take place.

So many plans and ideas, and seemingly not enough time or money to bring them to fruition!

Yet, the thoughts of animal care and husbandry that usually took up the majority of her mind slipped away before the first mile of her journey was behind her, replaced by a more troublesome matter.

Delano.

A rueful smile touched her lips as she considered that not very long ago all she'd wanted was for him to be gone, back to Trinidad, and out of her hair. Now, she actually dreaded his leaving.

It was a quandary, and she'd been avoiding giving it too much thought. But there was something about Delano that had opened her heart in a way no one else ever had.

Looking back on her relationship with Kyle, she could see where—emotionally struggling as she'd been then—she'd made herself an easy mark. After a lifetime of walking on eggshells and trying to navigate her mother's moods and whims, all he'd had to do was pretend to offer calm, stability and love, and she'd fallen into his arms.

She'd had no set boundaries, no barometer to gauge whether what she was experiencing was real or false. It had taken time and effort to examine herself, and build those parameters. And even her reaction to Delano's attempt to help the shelter showed there were still sore places in her psyche she needed to work on.

Not, she thought, because of Delano, but for her own sake. Because if the affair with Delano had taught her anything, it was that she still craved closeness and companionship. That life with him was far better than it had been before, or would be after he left.

Even now, having gone that far in her thinking, she couldn't bring herself to go the final step. To consider her true feelings for him—give them a name— would be too painful, in light of his imminent departure.

But she was just kidding herself. She'd realized how into him she was when she opened up to him about her mother, and Kyle. Not even Amity knew the full story, because Mellie couldn't bring herself to tell it. She'd gotten past the anger, but the shame lingered. Convincing herself she was a different, better, stronger person who didn't need to look back or tell anyone else what a fool she'd been had been easy.

She was about ten minutes out from Port Michael when her cell rang. It was Dr. Milo, so she answered it using the car's hands-free capability.

"Dr. Milo, how are you?"

"Mellie, have you seen Delano?"

Her heart stopped. She'd worked with the older man for years, and had never heard him sound anything but calm and cool. But now, although he was obviously trying to sound normal, there was tension in his voice.

"Not since about two thirty," she replied, trying to match his casual tone, although her heart rate was through the roof. "What's wrong?"

She heard Miss Eddie in the background, but couldn't make out what she was saying. Then Dr. Milo said, "It's probably nothing but I've been trying to reach him, and he's not answering his phone."

"I'm just outside Port Michael," Mellie said, forcing herself not to break the speed limit. Not by too much, anyway. "I'll check at the clinic, and let you know if he's there."

"Thank you, my dear. I… I'm sure he's fine."

"Did something happen to make you think otherwise?" It wasn't like Dr. Milo to fuss or go off half-cocked.

"No. No. Please don't worry. I'm sure he's fine," he repeated, but Mellie didn't believe him.

Skirting the edge of town saved her a few minutes and instead of going home, she went straight to the clinic. The relief she felt on seeing Delano's car still in the parking lot was immediate and immense.

After she'd parked, she rushed into the clinic, about to call his name when she heard the murmur of his voice from the office. Either he had someone with him, or was on the phone, so Mellie walked the few steps to the office, a sudden feeling of déjà vu making her pause at the door.

He wasn't hunting in the cupboard, as he had been the first night she saw him, but now, like then, he had his back to her.

"Yes," he said into the phone. "Nothing sooner? Okay, I'll take that."

Not wanting him to feel as though she were eavesdropping, Mellie stepped silently back out of the office and went down into the hospital area, turning on the lights as she went. There was a cat she didn't recognize, looking dazed and battered, one big golden eye blinking at her through the cage. Taking out the chart stuck in the holder, she read Delano's notes, and had just finished when she heard his footsteps in the corridor. They paused, and for a moment she thought he would leave without saying anything to her, but then she heard him striding toward where she was.

Clearly, Dr. Milo's behavior had rubbed off on her, making her paranoid. Of course, he wouldn't just take off once he realized she was there.

But then he stepped into the doorway and her heart sank, her expression freezing before the smile she was planning to send him could blossom.

He was pale, his complexion muddy, and although he was smiling it didn't reach his eyes, which looked at her with what seemed like blank indifference.

"I'm glad you're back," he said, and the distance she felt between them widened at the sound of his casual tone. "I wanted to tell you I'm leaving on Tuesday."

She couldn't answer, couldn't even ask him what was going on. Everything inside her was churning: brain, stomach, heart. Rendering her mute and unable even to move. Finally, after what felt like an age, she found her voice.

"What's happened?"

"Nothing," he said, but she heard the lie, even as he smiled again. "I need to get back to work. Dad's doing better. Aunt Eddie has everything under control. It's time."

"Okay." Inside she was screaming at herself to ask, *What about me? Us?* But the words stayed stuck in her head.

"I'll see you in the morning out in Grand Harbor. I'll get there for eight."

Mellie gathered herself then, pushing the hurt and shock down deep, drawing on every ounce of pride she could muster to nod, as if everything was normal.

Not falling down around her ears.

"Thanks," she replied, happy to have been able to keep her voice level. "See you then."

And when Delano walked away, she fought the urge to call him back, or run after him, even though it was what she most desperately wanted to do.

CHAPTER NINETEEN

DELANO WASN'T SURE how he got through Friday night but, somehow, he managed it.

Seeing Janice Gopaul had sliced his heart and soul into pieces again, and he wasn't sure he'd be able to put any of it back together.

As she stood there, unsmiling, he'd been thrown back in time. Suppressing the recollection of the last time he'd seen her, so he could speak to her normally and treat her dog, had taken everything he had inside.

He hadn't known she was back in St. Eustace. After Everard's death, she'd gone back to Guyana where she'd been born. No one had mentioned she'd returned, or was a client at the clinic and, he'd realized as they spoke, a board member of Mellie's shelter. Her sudden appearance had floored him, and brutally reminded him why he hated St. Eustace, and all the memories associated with it.

It also made him angry.

Why hadn't Mellie mentioned Mrs. Gopaul to him? Surely she knew their history, and would realize how devastating it would be for him to see her unexpectedly? Her failure to do so felt like betrayal and the worst type of cruelty.

He pled tiredness to his father and Aunt Eddie

and went to bed early, but couldn't help being aware of the worry in their eyes as they watched him. Yet, just like they had when he'd started seeing Mellie, they didn't comment or ask any questions, and he was thankful for it.

Lying in bed, staring at the ceiling, there was no way to stop the flow of memories.

Standing behind the almost closed door on the day of the funeral, hearing her voice from the living room, where she and Dad were.

"Someone should have stopped him," she'd said, in a hoarse furious tone that was forever etched in his mind. "Del should have, or you."

"Yes," Dad replied, so sadly and softly, Delano hardly heard him. "Yes."

But Dad hadn't been there, down by the water. Only Delano had known. Had seen Everard running into the surf.

Only Delano could have stopped him, but hadn't.

Had failed Everard, and Mum. Dad and Janice Gopaul.

And had paid for it, every day since.

Eventually, emotionally exhausted, he fell asleep, but woke up the next morning still weighed down with renewed sorrow and guilt.

The spay and neuter clinic was busy and bustling with vets, clients and volunteers. Thankfully, there was no sign of Janice, although she'd mentioned it to him when he'd seen her at the clinic.

It was easy to avoid Mellie, but Delano was constantly aware of where she was at all times. She didn't search him out, nor did she go out of her way to ignore him, but on the few occasions when they had reason to talk, she treated him with the same cool contempt she had when he'd first arrived.

It should have hurt, but there was a barrier between him and all emotion that couldn't be breached.

Sunday morning dawned overcast and drizzly, and suited his mood perfectly. Baldur hadn't left his side since Friday night, staring at him with questioning eyes, and lying as close as possible whenever Delano settled anywhere. Despite the dreary weather, Delano took the dog for a run as usual, but even a punishing, wet five miles did nothing to improve his mood or break him out of his emotional bubble.

As he was getting out of the shower, Aunt Eddie knocked on the door.

"Delano, your phone has been ringing nonstop. It might be important."

"Thanks," he called back, toweling off.

It went off again as he walked into his bedroom, and he picked it up. Not recognizing the number, he was a little brusque when he answered.

"Hello?"

"Dr. Logan?"

"Yes."

"Is Chappie Robinson, Doc, from up Preacher's Mount. We have a jackass caught down in a hole, and we trying to get him out. Dr. Mellie said to call you because you the best horse vet around."

At the sound of Mellie's name, something shivered to life inside, and Delano said, without hesitation, "I'll come up. Where are you?"

He rushed out of the house, leaving Baldur behind, followed by Aunt Eddie's grumbling about his not having breakfast yet, and how he'd catch his death in this weather. His anxiety was rising, breaking through the wall that had come down around him just days before, and he drove as quickly as he could on the slick roads.

Donkeys, like people, came with all different types of temperaments. Depending on whether the animal was hurt or not, the size of the hole and its depth, whoever took on the task of going down into it could be in danger.

And he had no doubt in his mind that if there was anyone in the hole, it would be Mellie.

If she was even on-site.

The sudden realization that the man he'd spoken to hadn't actually said Mellie was there brought such a rush of relief, Delano felt lightheaded for an instant.

But when he got to the site, that relief turned out to be misplaced.

Mellie was very much down in the hole, which was about six feet deep and perhaps eight across, with the frightened animal. She was damp and muddy, and utterly lovely, even while standing in inches of mud.

Without a second thought, he swung himself over the rim and landed next to her, squelching into the ankle-deep mud and making the donkey jerk against the rope halter Mellie was holding.

"Delano, you made it."

How incredibly calm she sounded, while his heart was trip-hammering in his chest, and his mouth was dry with fear.

"I'll take over down here," he said, when he could get the words out. Then he gestured to the men standing above them, around the hole. "Why don't you climb out and direct them as to what to do?"

The look she gave him was scornful and amused.

"Do you know me at all? I've already sent for straps, and one of the men has gone to see if his cousin can bring his bulldozer. The only thing we can do is wait, and make sure the animal is okay."

"Both of us don't need to do that." It felt imperative to get her out of danger...to safety. "I can manage on my own."

She didn't even bother to reply to his words.

Instead, she said, "Take a look at his left front cannon. I think it's hurt."

Resigned to her not budging, he replied, "Better to wait until we get him out of here. If he's in pain and I touch the area, he might kick."

"Or bite," Mellie said, clearly not too worried at the prospect. "I do say, though, he's one of the calmest donkeys I've had to work with, although I know that could change at any time."

Especially since the beast was, at that very moment, rolling its eyes at Delano, while its nostrils twitched.

There was a shout from above, and the earth beneath them rumbled.

"Shorty bring the excavator, Dr. Mellie. And he has the straps too."

After a few more minutes of what sounded like confusion above, a different man stuck his head over the side, and surveyed the scene.

"Dr. Mellie," he said, then twisted his mouth to the side. "What you want me to do?"

"You think you can hoist him up with the bulldozer, Shorty, if we get two straps under him?"

Another few seconds went by as Shorty's mouth twisted from side to side, and his eyes roamed the hole, the donkey and then the ground around the hole.

"I have to bring the dozer close up, and as long as the ground holds it that can work."

"Good. Tie the straps onto the bucket, and let's get this done."

Before Delano could object, Shorty disappeared.

"Did you hear what he said, Mellie?" Delano realized he was holding on to her arm in a too-tight grip, and forced himself to let go. "He's not even sure the ground around the hole can hold the weight of the bulldozer."

She shook her head. "If he was worried, he wouldn't agree to do it. Shorty is one of the best bulldozer operators on the island."

The rumbling of the engine got louder, and the donkey shifted nervously as the ground vibrated. Then the bulldozer bucket appeared, a man standing in it, holding the straps that had been tied onto the teeth.

Delano held up his hands, prepared to catch the strips of webbing, and the donkey brayed and bucked.

"Whoa, now." He could hardly hear Mellie over the racket. "You're okay. Don't go crazy on me now."

Laser-focused on getting them all out of the situation as quickly as possible, Delano passed the first strap under the donkey's belly, just behind the front legs. When he realized the strap wasn't long enough to be thrown back up to the bucket, he gestured for the bucket to be lowered farther, and the man above them passed the request on to Shorty.

After what felt like a year, he got both straps positioned, with Mellie too busy trying to calm the distressed animal to help.

When he shouted for the bulldozer bucket to be lifted, all he could do was hope the donkey wouldn't freak out, and kick itself out of the straps before it was back on solid ground.

Mellie was on one side of the animal's head, while Delano was on the other, both watching and keeping out of the way of the hind legs, as the donkey started rising out of the hole. It was still braying, like it was being murdered rather than rescued, but thankfully kept relatively still.

Delano had just let out the breath he'd been holding, when a shout rang out.

"Watch out! Watch out!"

The timbre of the bulldozer's engine changed, and the bucket swung to one side, sending the donkey swinging, just as the side of the hole gave way and a cascade of mud rushed in. Delano shouted with fear, as Mellie disappeared under it.

Mellie had felt the shifting of the earth behind her and, although bogged down in the mud at the bottom of the hole, had the chance to move one leg forward as the mud pushed her over. Although she went down on her knee, hard, the landslide didn't have a chance to engulf her, and she was in no real danger.

Not that you'd know it from Delano's reaction.

He went nuts, using his hands to try to free her, even when some of the other men jumped down with shovels and made quick work of it. Someone lowered in a ladder, and in short order they were out of the hole, although caked in mud.

Chappie came over, all smiles.

"That fool jackass. As soon as we take off the straps, him take off down back to him pasture. Thanks, you hear?"

"Get your fence fixed, Chappie," Mellie told him. "I'm not coming back up here to rescue him again."

"Yes, Dr. Mellie. I will."

The men were moving away in twos and threes, and the bulldozer had been shut off, and Shorty was walking over to join a group. Mellie was aware of Delano standing close beside her, but hesitated to turn to him.

She hadn't gotten over his behavior on Friday, and then yesterday at the spay and neuter event, when he hardly even looked her way. And when he did, it was as though they were strangers.

In the depths of Friday night, as she lay awake, determined not to cry over him, she'd admitted to herself just how much she felt for him. In her mind, it was too soon to call it love. Or maybe she just didn't really know what love looked like, to make the comparison. All she knew was that the end of their relationship had left a hole in her she wasn't sure would ever be filled.

What she really wanted was to walk away, to pretend he was already gone.

But he'd helped her just now, and shown concern in a way that told her he cared for her, even if it wasn't enough for him to be honest about how much, or why he was acting the way he was.

Mellie was fair-minded enough to at least thank him.

She turned, looking up at him, finding his gaze fixed on her. But it was the blank, shocked expression on his face that made her breath catch in her throat.

"Delano."

He blinked, but otherwise didn't react, like a sleepwalker, she thought. And when she put her hand on his arm, she realized he was shivering.

Impossible to leave him this way. He was in no condition to drive, and Mellie knew she'd rather take care of him than leave him to his own devices when he was obviously in some kind of distress.

"Come on," she said quietly, tugging his arm until he started walking with her toward her car. Thankfully, none of the other men seemed to notice anything unusual, since they were still chatting and laughing amongst themselves.

Getting him into the car, she quickly jumped in as well and started it.

As she bumped down the farm track toward the main road, she was trying to figure out how best to handle the situation. If she took him back to his father's house in this state, it might upset Dr. Milo.

Besides, if she was honest, she wanted to be the person to take care of him, to find out why he had reacted this way. It might also be a chance to figure out what had happened between them.

She was resigned to their affair having ended, but it would be nice to know why he'd done a one-eighty without any kind of explanation.

Getting to the house, she was relieved when Delano opened the car door himself and got out to walk with her to the back door. Before going inside, he even took off his mud-encrusted shoes; a sure sign he was coming out of whatever funk he'd fallen into at the rescue site.

Then he wandered over to the small kitchen table and sat heavily in a chair. Mellie followed, and took the seat across from him. When he reached for her hand, she didn't hesitate to take it.

"You scared me, Mellie." His voice was rough,

the timbre raw and pain filled. "When I saw the hole collapsing…"

His fingers tightened almost painfully, but Mellie didn't pull away.

"But I'm fine, Delano." She didn't add that in her opinion he was overreacting. She'd never make light of his distress that way. "You can relax now."

He shook his head, his gaze never leaving hers.

"It was my fault you were almost hurt. I should have protected you. Stopped you from staying down in there."

"You're not thinking straight." There was no sugarcoating it. "You couldn't have stopped me. I do what I need to, to help and rescue animals. That's who I am, and no one tells me what I can and can't do."

"Not even someone who loves you?"

CHAPTER TWENTY

THERE WAS ANGUISH in his words, and for a moment Mellie couldn't answer. There was too much in his question to fully comprehend. Before she could articulate her confusion, Delano continued speaking.

"I know I messed up the other night, walking away from you, but I realized today, when you were in danger, how much I love you."

Her heart was racing, joy flooding her, but Mellie knew there was something missing from his story.

"Why did you walk away, Delano?" His mouth tightened, as though in pain, and she knew she was on the right track. "What happened on Friday?"

He got up abruptly, releasing her hand. For a moment she thought he was going to walk away, but instead he paced across the kitchen, as though the effort to sit still was too much for him. He stopped at her kitchen window, his hands gripping the edge of her sink.

"Do you know how my mother died?" he asked, surprising Mellie with what sounded at first like a change of subject.

"Yes," she replied, stiffening, her hands clenched so tightly her fingers ached.

He'd only once ever spoken about his mother.

"The boy she was trying to save was my best friend, Everard."

"I know," she admitted.

"Mum and Dad had taken us to the beach." He spoke quietly, but with a gravelly edge, the words seeming to come reluctantly from his throat. "Mum was laying out the food. Dad went back to the car for something, and told us not to go into the water until he got back, because the sea was rough."

Mellie's hands tightened into fists, until her short nails were digging into her palms. She wanted to tell him to stop, not to relive the pain, but knew he needed to. And he needed her to listen.

Just like she'd needed to share her pain and embarrassment with him.

"Everard…" He paused, shaking his head. "Everard wasn't afraid of anything. He said he was going swimming, dared me to go with him. I wouldn't. I told him that if my father said not to swim until he got back, that's what I would do. I tried telling him that he wouldn't have to wait long, but he just laughed and ran into the water. There was a rip current and an undertow."

"I'm sorry." How inadequate those words sounded, but it was the best she could do through the lump in her throat.

"When he first called for help, I thought he was kidding, and shouted for him to stop. Mum ran down and dove in. Then, just as she got to him, they both disappeared."

He stopped, and swallowed. There was no need

for him to continue. Mellie could imagine the scene. The chaos and attempted rescue. The devasting news being delivered to not one but two families. The fear and guilt a little boy would feel at witnessing the death of two people he loved. With jerky movements he paced back across the kitchen and dropped into the chair again.

"You asked me what happened on Friday? Everard's mother came into the clinic. I hadn't seen her since just after the funerals. Since I heard her blame me for Everard's death." He shook his head slowly, then his expression changed from sorrow to a kind of desperate determination. "Now you know why I can't stay here. The memories come at me when I least expect them, and I know whenever Daddy looks at me, it must bring it all back for him, as well."

Oh, she could hardly bear to see his agony, but, at the same time, she couldn't leave him wallowing. She knew how detrimental it was to live in the past, castigating yourself without end.

"Delano." She sought the words, said a little prayer that she would get this conversation right. "Whatever Janice said to make you believe she blamed you, was said in the midst of the type of pain that would make anyone lash out. It's not something you can ever forget, but don't you think it's time to forgive yourself—and Janice—and put it behind you?"

"I don't blame her. How can I? She was right.

They died because I didn't stop Everard from going swimming. If I had—"

"How would you have stopped him?" The question popped out of her mouth before she even thought. "You said he wasn't afraid of anything. Was he the kind of child you could stop when he made up his mind to do something?"

Even in distress, Delano couldn't help the upward twitch of his lips. "Not him. He was adventuresome and hardheaded. Even his mother said so, more times than I could count, after we'd gotten into some scrape or other."

Mellie got up then and moved close to him, looking down into his face, willing him to listen to what she had to say.

"You've been living in the past. Beating yourself up for something that wasn't your fault and you couldn't have stopped even if you'd tried. And you know what breaks my heart, Delano?" When he shook his head, she said, "It's the thought that you could have died that day too. That I might never have had the chance to know and love you."

"Mellie."

Her name came out of him like a breath, almost too quiet to be heard, but the wonder and joy in it made Mellie's heart leap and race.

Then he was on his feet, holding her close, and it felt exactly like coming home.

"Come back with me," he said. "To Trinidad. You can start a shelter there. God knows there are enough stray animals to keep you busy."

And her heart, which had been sent soaring by his declaration of love, plummeted.

For a long moment she stayed where she was, her arms tight around his waist, her cheek pressed into the curve of his neck. Savoring his touch. His love.

When she pulled back to look up at him, her desolation must have shown, because the hope and joy in his expression faded.

"I can't do that, Delano." She said it softly, aching with the need to comfort him, but also with the determination to speak her truth. "This is my home. Where I've built a life for myself, found a place where I belong and can make a difference."

"But you can do that in Trinidad too." The note of desperation in his voice tore at her heart. "With me."

"I don't know that I can." She held Delano's gaze, as his eyes widened and his lips firmed into a straight line. "Even if I put aside everything I've worked for, abandoned my father and yours—just when Dr. Milo most needs someone to depend on— I'm not sure our relationship would work."

He released her, and stepped back, leaving her to shiver with the chill filling her center.

"I don't understand. Explain."

There was no plea in his voice, only demand. Anger, she suspected might come later, but for now he was shocked and hurt. Only honesty would do.

"The losses you suffered when you were young are horrendous, something you will never completely get over. But you've blamed yourself for that loss—*for twenty years*—and, as far as I can see, run away from every reminder of what happened. Every reminder of your mom and Everard, who were both so important to you. You've even run away from your father, who loves you so much and needs you now, and I'm sure needed you long before now too."

She could see his face tightening, his eyes going flat, but she couldn't stop now. Not when everything she wanted was at stake.

"If something were to happen—something bad—I got sick, or we lost a child, or I was hurt, would you run away from me too?"

He flinched, as though she'd struck him, and his face paled.

Had she gotten through to him, or would this be the end?

Delano shook his head, and anguish flashed across his face, then was hidden as he turned away. She saw his chest expand on a huge breath, and she waited for his response, the air pent in her own lungs.

"I don't know."

As his words registered, all sensation left her legs, and Mellie blindly reached for the back of the nearest chair, holding on to it for support. Her mouth was dry, and the thumping of her heart was harsh, made her feel sick.

Then she found her courage, and strength, and although she knew the pain of loss was hovering, waiting to swamp her, she straightened. When she reached out to touch his shoulder his muscles were locked and tight.

"Figure that out, Delano," she said, proud of how steady her voice came out. "Figure it out and let me know."

And when he strode out the door, she let him go.

Delano made his way out to the road, and stood there for a moment, lost. Mentally and emotionally battered.

And angrier than he could remember being for a long time.

How could Mellie not understand?

She was the first person he'd spoken to about what had happened all those years ago, what he'd seen and heard. Why couldn't she comprehend that he couldn't stay here, in this place so full of memories and reminders that crept out of doors or jumped out around corners?

That the pain of it was something he couldn't wait to get away from?

The rage boiling inside him was preferable to any other emotion just then, and it sustained him long enough for him to call a taxi to take him back to his car. In fact, he nurtured the anger, welcomed it, stewed in it all the way to his father's house.

But once there, he turned off the car and sat in it without getting out, reliving all Mellie had said, unable to sustain his fury.

Knowing she was right.

He had run away.

It had been the only thing he'd known to do, to deal with the agony of loss.

His entire world had fallen apart, and he still didn't know how to put it together again.

Wasn't sure he even wanted to try.

There was another world, removed from all of this, waiting for him back in Trinidad and it would be simpler—easier—to go back to it. Leave all this turmoil behind.

Finally, he got out of the car and made his way into the house, standing for a moment in the formal living room, which hardly ever got used.

It's for when visitors come, his mum used to say; a sentiment echoed by Aunt Eddie.

All of his mother's knickknacks were still on the shelves, and in the cabinets. The paintings she'd collected on the wall. He wouldn't be surprised if the rug was the same as it had been twenty years before too.

While he'd run away, his father seemed to have stayed stuck.

How had he been able to bear it?

Suddenly, it was imperative to know, and Delano went through to the patio, looking across to where his father sat beneath the shade of the poinciana tree.

Dad was leaning back in his chair, his eyes closed, and Delano hesitated, not wanting to disturb him if he was asleep. But before he could go back inside, Dad opened his eyes and smiled.

"Hi, son. Were you looking for me?"

The carefully searching way his father looked at him spoke volumes. Very little got past Dr. Milo and, although he hadn't commented, Delano knew his dad had noticed the change in him since Friday.

Suddenly, Delano was overtaken by waves of love and gratitude, sadness and longing.

Love for one of the best men he knew.

Gratitude for the fact that man was his father.

Sadness for the lost years, and an overriding longing to have them back.

Or, he thought, as he crossed the lawn to sit on the grass at his father's feet, longing to have the relationship they'd had before back, rather than the years.

The future doesn't have to be like the past...

Mellie had said it, in a variety of ways, and she was right.

Of course she was.

Looking up at his father, who was still and silently waiting, Delano felt as though perhaps Dad was feeling the same way too, and something inside him cracked open.

Never to be repaired.

"Dad…" It was a hoarse whisper, and he couldn't clear his throat enough to make it any clearer. "I want to talk to you about Mum—and the day she died."

And his father's nod, along with the hand he laid on Delano's shoulder, was everything he needed right then.

CHAPTER TWENTY-ONE

MELLIE DIDN'T KNOW whether she'd see Delano again, and refused to allow herself to speculate.

He'd been gone for half an hour before she'd collected herself enough to remember he hadn't had his car, but when she'd driven up to the farm where they'd rescued the donkey, his vehicle was no longer there.

Their conversation ran around and around in her mind, as she finally showered off the mud she'd accumulated during the donkey rescue, but she was sure there was nothing she could have done differently.

She loved Delano. More than she'd ever thought she'd love anyone. But she couldn't and wouldn't love blindly. That was the old Mellie; the one who would do anything to hold on to another's affection and attention, putting her own needs last, even when it was to her detriment.

How could she, in good conscience, abandon Dr. Milo, the clinic and her rescue? Especially when she wasn't one hundred percent sure of Delano's feelings.

He'd said he loved her but then, in the next minute, assumed the life she'd built for herself could and would be discarded without a second thought. No discussion necessary.

While there was a part of her that wanted to run away with him—go wherever he demanded—that wasn't healthy. Not for her, and definitely not for him.

There were deeper issues he needed to deal with, to be honest with himself about, before they had any chance of a real, lasting relationship.

It had taken him thinking she was in danger to even admit to his feelings for her and talk to her about the past. While Mellie had opened up to him, telling him things she'd never told anyone else, he'd been carefully curating what he shared with her. Keeping parts of himself—really important parts—locked away, and out of reach.

Needing something to keep her hands busy, Mellie dragged herself out into the cattery and started cleaning. Sheba came with her, much to the delight of the kittens, who acted as though the little dog was nothing more or less than put on the earth for their entertainment. Yet, Mellie couldn't even find joy in their antics. She wanted to cry, to scream, but couldn't.

She was frozen inside, waiting for the pain to hit.

When her phone buzzed, she almost ignored it, but habit had her looking at the screen, in case it was someone calling for a rescue.

It was from Delano, and Mellie's heart did a little flip as she stood for a moment without opening the message, trying to catch her breath. Exhaling deeply, she tapped the screen with her finger.

Meet me at Ludlow Beach, please.

Ludlow Beach? Wasn't that where his mother's accident had happened?

She didn't wait to change her clothes. Dressed in cutoff shorts and a stretched-out T, she hustled the dogs inside and rushed to the car.

The fifteen minutes it took to get there were some of the longest in her life, simply because she had no idea what to expect.

It was getting late, and since Ludlow Beach wasn't as popular as some of the others closer to Port Michael, there were few cars parked along the road. One of them belonged to Delano.

As she trotted down the path, which threaded its way through palms and sea grape trees, she could hear the sound of the ocean pounding on the nearby rocks. Coming out onto the beach itself, she looked up at the flagpole and her heart rate slowed when it was empty.

No red flag warning today.

Then she saw him, standing back from where the waves rolled up onto the shore, looking out over the water, his arms hanging down at his sides. The sun, low in the sky, limned him in golden light, emphasizing the breadth of his shoulders and the muscles of his legs, bare beneath the hem of his shorts.

She didn't know why, but she was cautious approaching him, and although her steps in the sand were soundless, before she got to him, he turned to look at her.

Then, he returned to gazing out to sea.

"I've never been back into the ocean, since that day," he said softly when she was standing beside him. "Dad says he hasn't either." He inhaled deeply, and shook his head. "We used to go sailing and fishing and of course swimming, all the time. I only just realized how much I miss it."

"I'm not surprised you stopped," she said, equally quietly. "What happened was traumatizing."

"It wouldn't be so bad if I'd been afraid for a while, even for a few years, and then got over it. But I allowed my fear to rule me. In that respect, and way too many others."

Mellie wanted to pull him close and tell him everything would be fine, but held back. Maybe all he needed was to talk, to get it all out, so he could move forward, with or without her.

"I didn't want to let anyone close." He said it in such a matter-of-fact way, he could have been talking about the weather. "Not Dad or Aunt Eddie, definitely not my ex-wife. When you let people in, they have the power to hurt you. To turn your life upside down, and tear out your heart."

"That's true," she agreed, aching for him—for the boy who'd learned too young the pain of loss.

"But they also have the power to heal, if you let them in. I spoke to Dad." Mellie's little gasp of surprise and pleasure couldn't be suppressed, but she didn't know if he'd even heard it. "We talked about Mum, and Everard, and what happened here that day. And what happened afterward too. I think... I think it was good for us both."

"I'm so glad, Delano." And she was, wholeheartedly. "For both of you."

He turned to her then, cupping her cheeks so he could meet and hold her gaze. "For the first time in a long time, I feel as though happiness is within my reach, Mellie. But it won't be complete without you. Will you give me another chance? Let me show you how much I love you, and value you and all that you do? Make it up to you for trying to use our love to coerce you into making a choice you didn't want to?"

How could she say no to that?

"Yes." Reaching up, she kissed him gently, before repeating, "Yes."

He smiled, his face and eyes lighting up, all his love in full display in his expression.

"We have options," he said, rushing the words, as though wanting her to know he meant what he said. "Dad has offered us both the clinic, in equal share, as long as he can consult and come in a few days a week. Or you can concentrate mostly on the rescuing and educational work, and work part-time at the clinic. Or—"

Mellie shut him up by kissing him again, thoroughly. So that by the time their lips parted, they were both breathless and aroused.

Somehow she found the breath to say, "We'll talk about it, and decide. Together. Later."

Picking her up, Delano swung her around, then put her back down to bend and unlace his sneakers.

"Come on," he said. "Come into the water with me."

And she was crying with joy as they walked into the sea together, leaving fears behind on the shore. Swimming toward the future, and into an ocean of love.

EPILOGUE

MELLIE SAT ON a stool outside the stable door, smiling and shaking her head.

"Now I remember why I didn't specialize in large animal medicine," she said.

Delano looked over at her and chuckled as he removed the arm-length disposable glove he'd worn to reposition the foal prior to delivery.

"It's not too bad, once you get used to it," he said, shrugging off the surgical gown.

"And with this result, it's all worth it," her father added. He was gently wiping the bay foal down with handfuls of straw, while the mare, Marmalade, sniffed and snuffled her new colt.

"He *is* awfully cute," Mellie conceded.

"And it's just as well I'm the one Mr. Charlie called to deliver him." Delano gave her a pointed look over his shoulder as he washed his hands. "You could belly up to the mare, but your arm would be too short."

Mellie stuck out her tongue at him, even while acknowledging he was right.

Being thirty-nine weeks pregnant did make it difficult to get too close to anything!

"Speaking of which," her father interjected, "aren't you supposed to be resting?"

It was a mark of her father's concern for his mare that he was just bringing it up, and Delano snorted in response, earning himself a narrow-eyed glare from his wife.

"I'm on maternity leave," she replied, wondering how many more times she'd have to say it. "Not bed rest. The doctor said to keep active, just not to overdo it. Sitting here watching you two—and Marmalade—do all the work isn't exactly stressful."

"Aunt Eddie has already texted me three times this morning," Delano groused to his father-in-law, while drying his hands. "And Dad isn't much better. I don't dare tell them she isn't at home with her feet up."

Mellie snorted, but the warm sense of contentment she felt at his words was undeniable.

She and Delano had been together almost three years, and the time had flown by in a whirlwind of experiences. Through their marriage and taking over of the clinic, as well as arranging freedom flights for dogs and expanding the shelter, they'd lived, worked, laughed, teased and grown together.

And, most of all, loved.

So much loving that she couldn't picture her world or life without him.

For the first time ever Mellie felt truly secure, surrounded by family and friends, with Delano always by and on her side. And with their baby due any day now, who could ask for more?

"Let me get you home, babe," Delano said, coming over and holding out a hand to help her up. "Maybe stop and get you some ice cream on the way?"

"That would be perfect."

Taking his hand, she stood and was enfolded in his arms, where she longed always to be.

Safe.

Happy.

Home.

* * * * *

If you enjoyed this story, check out these other great reads from Ann McIntosh

The Nurse's Holiday Swap
Twin Babies to Reunite Them
Christmas Miracle on Their Doorstep
One-Night Fling in Positano

All available now!

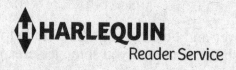

HARLEQUIN
Reader Service

Enjoyed your book?

Try the perfect subscription for Romance readers and get more great books like this delivered right to your door.

See why over 10+ million readers have tried Harlequin Reader Service.

Start with a Free Welcome Collection with free books and a gift—valued over $20.

Choose any series in print or ebook. See website for details and order today:

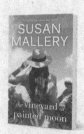
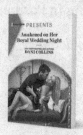
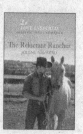
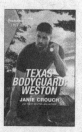

TryReaderService.com/subscriptions